Emergency Medical Procedures for the

The procedures in this book have been developed in consultation with:

Gordon A. Benner, MD
Chairman, Medical Subcommittee of the
Outing Committee, Sierra Club

Richard E. Church, MD
Leadership Chairman, Worcester
Chapter, Appalachian Mountain Club

Lance Feild
President, International Backpackers
Association

Menasha Ridge Press
Birmingham, Alabama

Outdoor activities are assumed risk sports. While every effort has
been made to insure that the information in this book is accurate
and reflects current practice, first aid and emergency procedures
change constantly. This book is intended as a guide and cannot be
expected to replace an approved and appropriate course in first aid,
CPR or emergency procedures.

Originally published as *Emergency Medical Procedures for the
Backpacker*, © 1979 Patient Care Publications, Inc.

Copyright© 1987 Patient Care Publications, Inc.
All rights reserved.
Art/Design: Tom Fowler
Art Revisions: Cori Inglis
Editor: Nicole Jones
Production: Nancy Burleson
Manufactured in the United States of America
ISBN 0-89732-051-4

Library of Congress Cataloging-in-Publication Data

Emergency medical procedures for the backpacker.
    Emergency medical procedures for the outdoors.

    Reprint. Originally published: Emergency medical procedures for
the backpacker. Darien, CT: Patient Care Publications, Special
Publications Group, c1979.
        1. Backpacking—Accidents and injuries—Outlines, syllabi,
etc.   2. First aid in illness and injury—Outlines, syllabi, etc. 3.
Medical emergencies—Outlines, syllabi, etc. I. Benner, Gordon
A. II. Church, Richard E., 1920-   . III. Feild, Lance, 1927-
    . IV. Title.   (DNLM: 1. Camping—popular works.   2.
Emergencies—popular works.   3. First Aid.
WA 292 E532 1979a]
RC88.9.H55E46   1987   616.02'52'0247965   87-18508
ISBN 0-89732-051-4 (pbk.)

Menasha Ridge Press
3169 Cahaba Heights Road
Birmingham, AL 35243

Introduction

These emergency medical procedure charts have been designed to help you handle potentially dangerous or troublesome situations that may occur while backpacking or camping. The chart on page 1 reviews how to prepare for a safe trip. The contents on p. **iii** will quickly refer you to the specific problem. When a situation calls for you to get help, the section beginning on p. 46 will help you decide whether a person with a specific medical problem is able to walk for help or whether he should be left alone and gives the precautions to take for each alternative. Make-do medical supplies not suggested in the list of basic first aid supplies are detailed in charts where appropriate. For example, a fracture might call for a sling and/or a splint. Suggestions on how to make these from materials you are carrying or that are close at hand are on the medical procedure chart.

Remember that the key to first aid is prevention: being in good shape, following a healthy diet, and taking enough well-fitting clothes designed to offer plenty of protection against the elements — cold, heat, sun, and precipitation. Hypothermia caused by exposure to rain and wind is not uncommon even in warm weather. Similarly, heat exhaustion may occur after strenuous activity even in cool weather.

When a medical emergency occurs:

Remain calm. Take a deep breath, then read these instructions. With all emergencies, except when there is no pulse (then turn immediately to CPR, pp. 5-7), one or two minutes spent getting the situation under control will improve your effectiveness.

Look up the major problem in the Contents. Before doing anything, read over the chart you'll be using to become familiar with the recommended procedures and equipment. If a serious emergency occurs that is not listed, the best procedure is to radio for help, send a distress signal (see below), or go for help (after setting up a shelter for the victim and leaving food and water). If you must leave the person alone, be sure to mark your trail (see next page).

Provide only emergency care outlined in these charts unless you receive instructions for additional care from a medically trained person via radio or other means.

Use common sense with these charts; only you know your particular situation. The primary rule of emergency aid is to cause no further injury. Most important during any medical emergency — Remember your ABCs:

— Make sure the *airway* is unobstructed.
— Make sure the person is *breathing*.
— Be sure the *circulation* of blood is maintained.
   (Heart is kept pumping, bleeding is controlled, etc.)

Distress Signals

If you need assistance, use one or more of the following:

— Standard Ground-to-Air Signals: As large as possible, illustrate by digging in sand or snow or use tree limbs, rocks, clothing, etc. Be sure the symbols contrast the ground color as much as possible.

   ■   for "Require doctor — serious injuries"
   ■■   for "Require medical supplies"

— Universal Distress Signals: A series of three sights or sounds, such as shouts, blows on a whistle, high-frequency beeps, gunshots, or flashes of light.

— SOS Morse Code Distress Signal: A series of three dots, three dashes, three dots made by blows on a whistle, high-frequency beeps, or flashes of light.

   · · · — — — · · · means SOS or Help!

Continued on next page

— A large flag at the top of a tree — the brighter, the better.
— A mirror or other shiny object flashed across the sky several times a day to attract planes.
— Flares

Marking Your Trail
Never leave someone who is injured without marking your trail with one or more of the following:
— branches
— mounds of rocks (cairns)
— arrows carved in the dirt
— grass tied in bunches
— sticks dug into the ground at the side of the trail
— torn pieces of cloth tied to branches
Use one of the above methods to mark your trail through snow; don't rely on footprints — more snow may fall or the snow may melt.

Contents

Contents

¹Before You Go

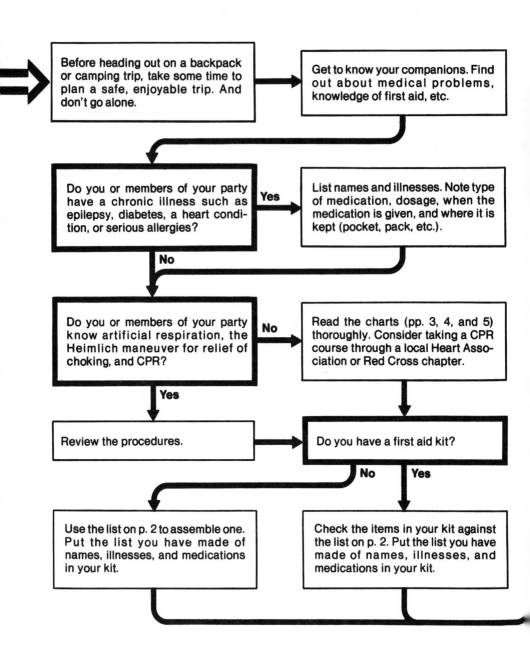

Before heading out on a backpack or camping trip, take some time to plan a safe, enjoyable trip. And don't go alone.

Get to know your companions. Find out about medical problems, knowledge of first aid, etc.

Do you or members of your party have a chronic illness such as epilepsy, diabetes, a heart condition, or serious allergies?

Yes

List names and illnesses. Note type of medication, dosage, when the medication is given, and where it is kept (pocket, pack, etc.).

No

Do you or members of your party know artificial respiration, the Heimlich maneuver for relief of choking, and CPR?

No

Read the charts (pp. 3, 4, and 5) thoroughly. Consider taking a CPR course through a local Heart Association or Red Cross chapter.

Yes

Review the procedures.

Do you have a first aid kit?

No   **Yes**

Use the list on p. 2 to assemble one. Put the list you have made of names, illnesses, and medications in your kit.

Check the items in your kit against the list on p. 2. Put the list you have made of names, illnesses, and medications in your kit.

Will children be accompanying you? — **Yes** → Go over the charts with them and explain how to get help if you are injured.

No

Will there be poisonous snakes in the area (see p. 36)? — **Yes** → Carry a snakebite kit. Suggest that everyone wear high boots.

No

Will there be poisonous spiders (Brown Recluse or Black Widow) or poisonous scorpions in the area (see p. 37)? — **Yes** → Encourage all members to shake out clothes, sleeping bags, and shoes before using and be careful about putting hands in rocky areas.

No

Check daily for ticks if the area is heavily infested.

Before any backpack or camping trip, tell at least one responsible person where you're going, when you'll be there, and how long you'll be gone. Be sure to let this person know if you change your plans. → Have a good, safe trip.

2 Basic Medical Supplies

Basic Medical Supplies for Use With the Emergency Medical Procedures for Backpackers.

The supplies specified are divided into two lists: one consists of medical supplies, which should be kept separate for emergency care and first aid; the other consists of cooking or basic supplies, which may be used for other purposes as well as for emergencies. The designated provisions include only those supplies required in these charts. Most of these items are available in supermarkets or pharmacies.

Although many more items could be included, weight and space are limited while backpacking. For this reason, medical supplies which come in large containers, such as rubbing alcohol, may be transferred to smaller, unbreakable containers. The required amounts depend upon the length of the trip. *Be sure to label every container.*

The two lists should meet the needs for treating injuries or illnesses most frequently encountered by backpackers. However, if anyone in your backpacking party has a history of allergic reaction to insect stings, or if your party is hiking in an area densely inhabited by insects, we recommend that you include an insect-bite kit, available by prescription from your physician. It is also advisable to take along a snake-bite kit if you will be backpacking in a region populated by poisonous snakes. If your party will be fishing, we recommend that you add wirecutters, pliers, or some other heavy-duty shearing device to the list. One item not listed is fresh water, which is required for a number of emergency situations. Be sure you carry a sufficient quantity for drinking and medical purposes.

Medical Supplies
activated charcoal tablets (medicinal)
adhesive tape (1 inch)
antacids (Gelusil, Maalox, Mylanta)
antihistamine/decongestant (Contac, Dristan, Sudafed)
aspirin and acetaminophen (Tylenol, Datril)
baking soda
calamine lotion
clean cloth (pieces of sheet)
cotton swabs
elastic bandage (3 inch)
emergency blanket ("space blanket", etc.)
Epsom salts (4 oz.)
fever thermometer
hydrogen peroxide
insect-bite kit*
lip balm (ChapStick, etc.)
oil of cloves
paraffin or candle
petroleum jelly (Vaseline, etc.)
razor blade
rubbing alcohol
scissors
smelling salts
snake-bite kit**
sterile gauze bandage (3 inch)
sterile gauze pads (4 x 4 inches)
syrup of ipecac
topical antibiotic ointment (Triple-Antibiotic Ointment, Neosporin, Bacitracin, etc.)
tweezers

Cooking and Basic Supplies that can be used as Medical Supplies
aluminum foil
bouillon cubes
cup
drinking water
fruit juices (powdered)
honey
hard candy
milk (powdered)
plastic bags
salt or salt tablets
soap (without deodorant, cold cream)
sugar
tea
rust-proof knife (stainless steel)

*If a member of party is allergic to stings.
**If hiking in an area inhabited by poisonous snakes.

³Artificial Respiration

This chart should only be used if the person is not breathing, but his heart is beating. Check the neck carefully for a carotid pulse; it may be very faint. If the person has no pulse, see *CPR* (p. 5). Artificial respiration should be performed even if a person has been under water for up to 60 minutes. If there is a possibility that the person choked before breathing stopped, see *Choking* (p. 4).

Clear airway. Remove foreign matter, using a cloth or tissue-wrapped finger if necessary.

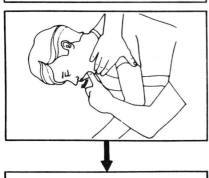

Use one hand to gently lift person's chin while tilting head back with other hand. **Do not tilt head if neck injuries are suspected.**

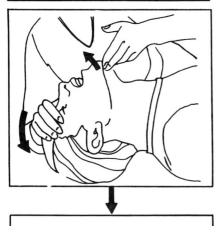

For an adult pinch nostrils with fingers of hand resting on forehead. Do not pinch nostrils of an *infant*.

Continue to tilt head, take a deep breath, and seal your mouth tightly around person's mouth or over nose and mouth for infants.

Give two full breaths. For infants, blow only small puffs of air. If the chest does not rise, make sure all foreign matter and secretions have been removed and that the head is correctly tilted, **unless neck injuries are suspected.**

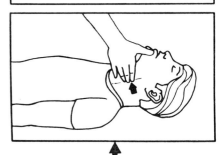

Feel the neck for a carotid pulse. If there is none, see *CPR*. (p. 5).

Continue ventilation for *adults* and *older children* at a rate of 12 inflations per minute — 20 for infants, checking carotid pulse every 3-4 minutes, until the person breathes regularly without assistance.

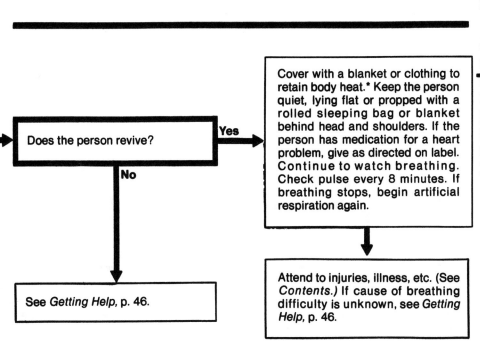

Does the person revive?

Yes

Cover with a blanket or clothing to retain body heat.* Keep the person quiet, lying flat or propped with a rolled sleeping bag or blanket behind head and shoulders. If the person has medication for a heart problem, give as directed on label. Continue to watch breathing. Check pulse every 8 minutes. If breathing stops, begin artificial respiration again.

No

See *Getting Help,* p. 46.

Attend to injuries, illness, etc. (See *Contents.)* If cause of breathing difficulty is unknown, see *Getting Help,* p. 46.

*If weather is very warm and person's skin does not feel cool and clammy, covering will not be necessary.

4 Choking
(Heimlich Maneuver)

Signs & Symptoms: *Clutching throat/initial coughing with gasping followed by inability to cough or speak/sudden loss of consciousness while eating and blue or gray skin, fingernails and mucous membranes.*

If the person has been injured, do not move unless necessary. Use appropriate method shown below to dislodge obstruction.

The person who is choking is:

A Small Child

Turn the child's head down over your arm, keeping the head lower than the body. Administer 4 sharp blows between the shoulder blades.

Has object been dislodged?

No

Yes

Child should be checked by a physician as soon as possible.

An Adult

Is the person conscious?

No

Yes

Wrap arms around person from behind. Make fist with one hand, covering it with the other. Place thumb side (top) of fist just above person's navel but below rib cage. Thrust fist upward and back into person's abdomen. Repeat this several times.

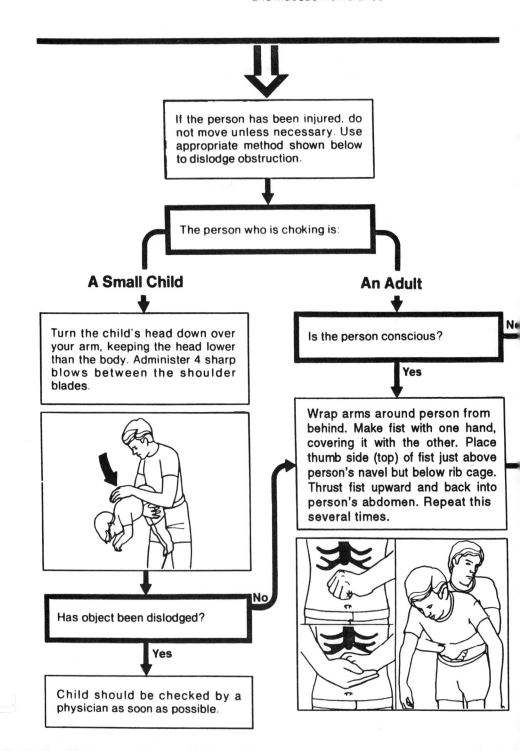

If person was not eating, clutches chest, or indicates there is extreme chest pain, see Chest Pain, p. 9.

Kneel astride person's hips. Cross flat hands and place slightly above navel, but below rib cage. Thrust heel of bottom hand into abdomen with quick upward thrusts. Repeat 6-10 times. (If person vomits, turn head to side.) Next, do a finger sweep with your index finger using a "hooking" action. Open airway using the chin lift/head tilt method (p. 3) and give two full breaths.

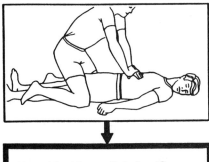

Has object been dislodged?

Yes → Person should be checked by a physician as soon as possible.

No

Try procedures again until the airway obstruction is cleared. If still no response, see "Getting Help", p. 46.

5 CPR
(1 rescuer)

For infants, see *CPR (Infants)*, p. 7.

If 2 or more rescuers, see p. 6. Begin CPR as soon as possible. Do not use CPR on a person whose heart is beating. It may cause serious complications. Check the neck artery carefully; pulse may be weak. If there is a heartbeat but no sign of breathing, see *Artificial Respiration*, p. 3.

Place person flat on back on ground. Ask "Are you all right?" two or three times. If person is not aroused, lightly shake or slap.

Kneel at side of head. Clear airway. Remove any foreign materials from mouth. Use one hand to lift chin while tilting head back with other hand. **Do not tilt head if neck injuries are suspected.**

Pinch nostrils together and rest palm of hand on forehead. Take a deep breath and seal your lips tightly over mouth. Blow 2 breaths, releasing mouth after each breath.

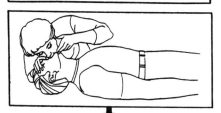

Feel pulse for 5-10 seconds. Check the neck artery carefully; pulse may be weak. If there is a pulse, but breathing is absent, continue only ventilation at a rate of 12 per minute until person revives.

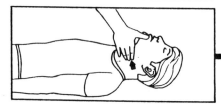

If no pulse, follow ribcage up to center of chest. Place index and middle finger on center of lower breastbone.

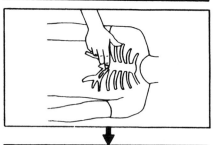

Place heel of other hand immediately next to and touching the index finger.

For adults, and children over 80 pounds only, place heel of the first hand directly over the wrist of the other hand on the person's lower breastbone. Clasp fingers and bend those of lower hand back. *For children under 80 pounds,* use only heel of one hand.

Lean directly over the person and straighten your arm(s).

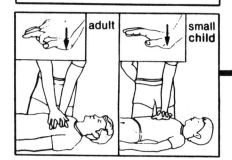

adult

small child

Use straight-down pressure through both arms (one arm for child under 80 pounds) to push breastbone against heart. *For an adult,* depress breastbone 1½" to 2"; *for a child,* ¾" to 1½".

The compression/relaxation combination is performed at a rate of 80 times per minute. Count one-and-two-and-three, etc. Completely release pressure during relaxation phase without lifting your hand(s) from person's chest.

After 15 compressions, breathe twice into the mouth. Repeat the 15-to-2 cycle 5 times.

Does the person revive?

No

Yes

Check breathing and neck pulse carefully. If no pulse, give two full breaths and continue the cycle with 15 chest compressions. Check pulse and breathing after every 5-10 cycles until the person is revived, help arrives, or you can no longer continue. If there is a pulse, but breathing is weak or absent, continue only ventilation at a rate of 12 per minute until the person revives.

Place the person in a sitting position and loosen clothing to relieve pressure. Keep person warm and check for continued breathing and pulse.

Attend to injuries, illness, etc. (See Contents.) If cause of cardiac arrest is unknown see *Getting Help,* p. 46.

6 CPR

(2nd rescuer trained in CPR)

For infants, see *CPR* (Infants), p. 7.

If another person trained in CPR is at the scene, the person should do two things: first, phone EMS for help if this has not been done; second, take over CPR when 1st person is tired.

Rescuer 2: Identify yourself as a person trained in CPR who is willing to help and phone EMS for help if that has not already been done. When the 1st rescuer is tired, take over after the 1st rescuer finishes the next set of two breaths.

Kneel beside the victim opposite of the 1st person, tilt victim's head using chin lift/head tilt method (p. 3), and feel the pulse for 5 seconds. Check the neck artery carefully; pulse may be weak. If there is a pulse, but breathing is weak or absent, continue only ventilation at a rate of 12 per minute until the person revives. **Do not give chest compressions on a person who has a pulse.**

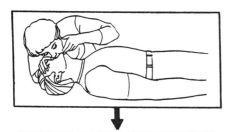

If no pulse, give 2 full breaths and continue the cycle with chest compressions (p. 5) at a rate of 80 per minute. After 15 compressions, breathe two full breaths into the mouth. Repeat this 15-to-2 cycle five times.

Rescuer 1: The 1st person should check the adequacy of the 2nd person's breathing and compressions. This is done by watching the chest rise and fall during rescue breathing, and by feeling the neck artery for an artificial pulse during chest compressions. The artificial pulse will tell you if blood is moving throughout the body.

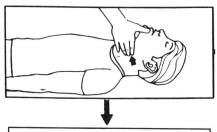

Check breathing and neck pulse carefully. If no pulse, give two full breaths and continue CPR with 15 chest compressions. Check pulse and breathing every 5-10 cycles until the person is revived, help arrives, or you can no longer continue. If there is a pulse, but breathing is weak or absent, continue only ventilation at a rate of 12 per minute until the person revives.

7 CPR
(Infants)

Begin CPR immediately. If 2 or more rescuers, 1 begin CPR while other gets help. Do not use CPR on an infant whose heart is beating: It may cause serious complications. Check carefully above left nipple for heartbeat; pulse may be weak. If there is a heartbeat but no sign of breathing, see Artificial Respiration, p. 3.

Place infant flat on back. Try to arouse by lightly shaking or tapping hard on bottom of foot.

Clear airway. Remove any foreign material from mouth and gently support neck with head slightly tilted. **Do not push head back at all if neck injuries are suspected.**

Seal your mouth over infant's mouth and nose and blow 2 small puffs of air.

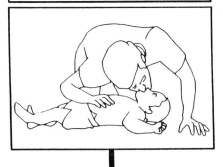

Feel for pulse at brachial artery (middle of inside upper arm) for 5-10 seconds. Check carefully; pulse may be weak. If there is a pulse, but breathing is weak or absent, continue only ventilation at a rate of 20 per minute until infant revives.

If no pulse, spread one hand over chest so that thumb is at base of throat and little finger is at end of breastbone. Keep index finger and middle finger together and lift others from chest.

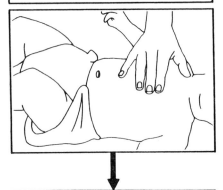

With tips of index finger and middle finger press gently on center of brestbone, depressing 1/2" to 3/4".

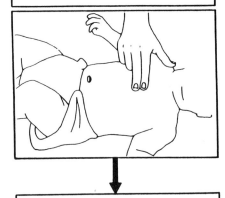

The compression/relaxation combination is performed at a rate of 80-100 times per minute. Count 1-2-3, etc.

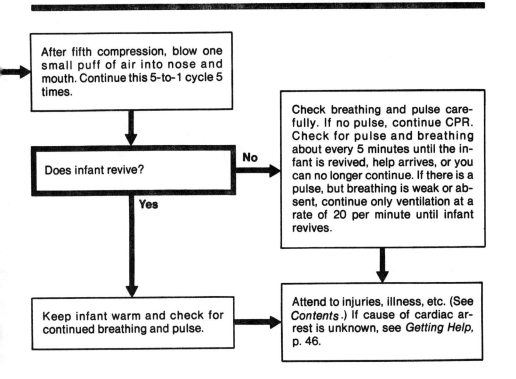

After fifth compression, blow one small puff of air into nose and mouth. Continue this 5-to-1 cycle 5 times.

Does infant revive?

No

Yes

Check breathing and pulse carefully. If no pulse, continue CPR. Check for pulse and breathing about every 5 minutes until the infant is revived, help arrives, or you can no longer continue. If there is a pulse, but breathing is weak or absent, continue only ventilation at a rate of 20 per minute until infant revives.

Keep infant warm and check for continued breathing and pulse.

Attend to injuries, illness, etc. (See *Contents*.) If cause of cardiac arrest is unknown, see *Getting Help*, p. 46.

8 Abdominal Pain

Abdominal pain should never be taken lightly. If the person has experienced this pain before, treat in same manner as previously. If pain continues or changes, continue through chart. Do not apply heat to abdomen. Keep person lying quietly.

Ask about or check for the following symptoms or conditions. Does the person have . . .

Sharp or burning pain in mid-upper abdominal region, with:
— pain radiating to arm(s), neck, or jaw?
— difficulty breathing?
— skin, lips, or nails pale or bluish?

Yes →
— Have person lie back with rolled blankets or sleeping bag behind head and shoulders.
— If this is a heart patient with medication, give medication as directed on label.
— Loosen clothing. Provide good ventilation. Cover with a blanket or clothing to retain body heat.*
— Continue to watch breathing. If it stops, see *Artificial Respiration,* p. 3.
— See *Getting Help,* p. 46.

No ↓

Sharp or burning pain in mid-upper abdominal region with none of the above?

Yes →
Problem may be indigestion, gastritis, or ulcer.
— Give antacids or milk.
— Do not give coffee, tea, alcohol, or aspirin-containing remedies for 24 hours.
If pain persists more than one hour or other symptoms occur, see *Getting Help,* p. 46.

If pain subsides, have person eat only light foods (soups, broths, etc.) for 24 hours, then gradually return to normal diet. If symptoms recur, seek medical care as soon as possible.

No ↓

Diabetes, with:
— flushed face?
— lethargy, drowsiness?
— hot, dry skin?
— deep, rapid breathing?
— fruity breath odor?

Yes →

See *Diabetic Emergencies,* p. 11.

No ↓

— Hard and rigid belly?
— Bloody or "coffee grounds" vomit with no recent abdominal injury?
— Bloody diarrhea?

Yes →
See *Getting Help,* p. 46.

No

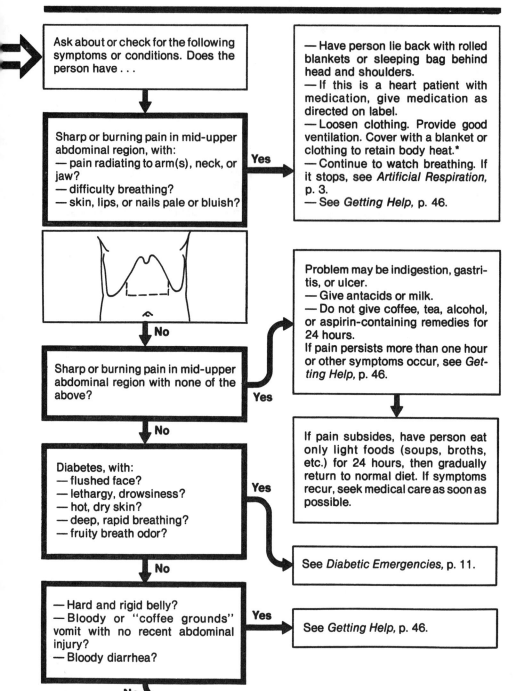

Calm the person by talking while attending to the problem. Explain what you are doing. Try not to show concern; act with confidence. Your calm behavior can help to reassure the sick person.

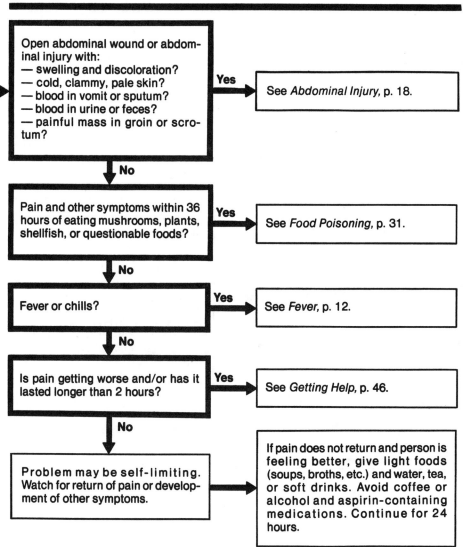

Open abdominal wound or abdominal injury with:
— swelling and discoloration?
— cold, clammy, pale skin?
— blood in vomit or sputum?
— blood in urine or feces?
— painful mass in groin or scrotum?

Yes → See *Abdominal Injury,* p. 18.

No ↓

Pain and other symptoms within 36 hours of eating mushrooms, plants, shellfish, or questionable foods?

Yes → See *Food Poisoning,* p. 31.

No ↓

Fever or chills?

Yes → See *Fever,* p. 12.

No ↓

Is pain getting worse and/or has it lasted longer than 2 hours?

Yes → See *Getting Help,* p. 46.

No ↓

Problem may be self-limiting. Watch for return of pain or development of other symptoms.

→ If pain does not return and person is feeling better, give light foods (soups, broths, etc.) and water, tea, or soft drinks. Avoid coffee or alcohol and aspirin-containing medications. Continue for 24 hours.

*If weather is very warm and person's skin does not feel cool and clammy, covering will not be necessary.

9 Chest Pain

Most chest pain is caused by indigestion or muscular strain. If it is severe, persistent, or worrisome, check symptoms below for more serious ailments.

Watch for breathing problems. If breathing stops, see *Artificial Respiration*, p. 3.

Did the person fall or get hit in chest?

Yes → See *Chest Injury*, p. 24.

No

Are the following symptoms present?
— intense, squeezing, constricting pain, possibly radiating (extending) to the neck, jaw, shoulders and/or arm(s)
— nausea and/or vomiting, cold sweats, difficulty breathing

Yes →

— Have person lie back with rolled blankets or sleeping bag behind head and shoulders.
— If this is a heart patient with medication, give medication as directed on label.
— Loosen clothing. Provide good ventilation. Cover with a blanket or clothing to retain body heat.*
— Continue to watch breathing. If it stops, see *Artificial Respiration*, p. 3.
— See *Getting Help*, p. 46.

No

Is the pain only in the mid-upper abdomen?

Yes → See *Abdominal Pain*, p. 8.

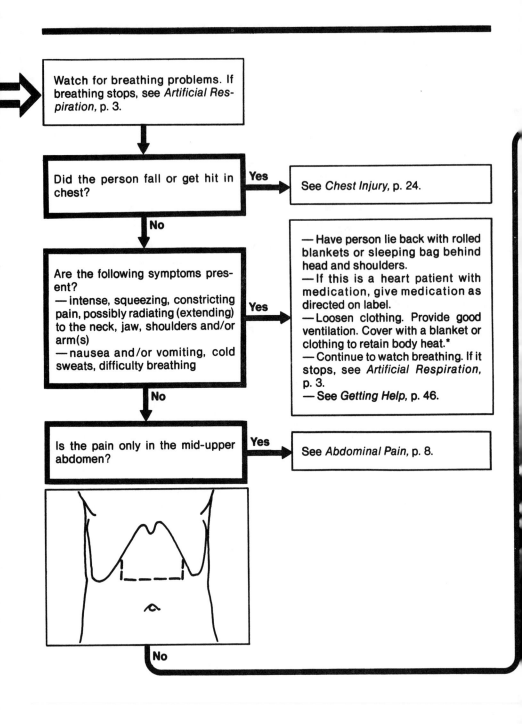

No

Calm the person by talking while attending to the problem. Explain what you are doing. Try not to show concern; act with confidence. Your calm behavior can help to reassure the sick person.

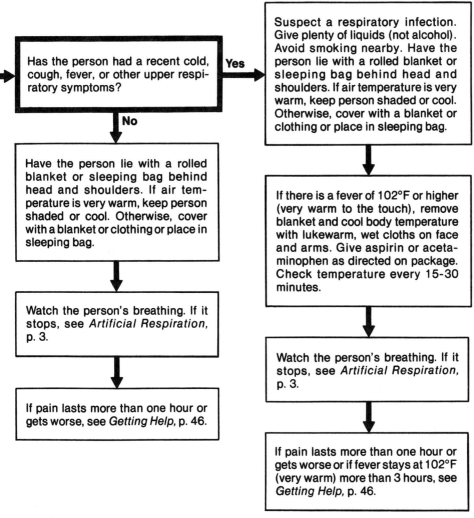

Has the person had a recent cold, cough, fever, or other upper respiratory symptoms?

Yes

Suspect a respiratory infection. Give plenty of liquids (not alcohol). Avoid smoking nearby. Have the person lie with a rolled blanket or sleeping bag behind head and shoulders. If air temperature is very warm, keep person shaded or cool. Otherwise, cover with a blanket or clothing or place in sleeping bag.

No

Have the person lie with a rolled blanket or sleeping bag behind head and shoulders. If air temperature is very warm, keep person shaded or cool. Otherwise, cover with a blanket or clothing or place in sleeping bag.

If there is a fever of 102°F or higher (very warm to the touch), remove blanket and cool body temperature with lukewarm, wet cloths on face and arms. Give aspirin or acetaminophen as directed on package. Check temperature every 15-30 minutes.

Watch the person's breathing. If it stops, see *Artificial Respiration*, p. 3.

Watch the person's breathing. If it stops, see *Artificial Respiration*, p. 3.

If pain lasts more than one hour or gets worse, see *Getting Help*, p. 46.

If pain lasts more than one hour or gets worse or if fever stays at 102°F (very warm) more than 3 hours, see *Getting Help*, p. 46.

*If weather is very warm and person's skin does not feel cool and clammy, covering will not be necessary.

10 Convulsion
(Including Epileptic Seizure)

Signs & Symptoms: *involuntary jerking of muscles/possible loss of bowel and bladder control/unconsciousness/cessation of breathing/gradual subsidence followed by semi-consciousness*

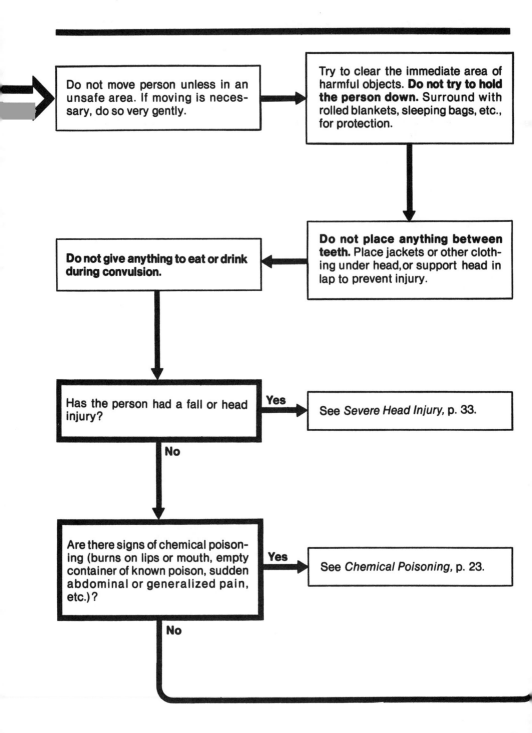

Do not move person unless in an unsafe area. If moving is necessary, do so very gently.

Try to clear the immediate area of harmful objects. **Do not try to hold the person down.** Surround with rolled blankets, sleeping bags, etc., for protection.

Do not place anything between teeth. Place jackets or other clothing under head, or support head in lap to prevent injury.

Do not give anything to eat or drink during convulsion.

Has the person had a fall or head injury?

Yes — See *Severe Head Injury*, p. 33.

No

Are there signs of chemical poisoning (burns on lips or mouth, empty container of known poison, sudden abdominal or generalized pain, etc.)?

Yes — See *Chemical Poisoning*, p. 23.

No

Calm the person by talking while attending to the problem. Explain what you are doing. Try not to show concern; act with confidence. Your calm behavior can help to reassure the sick or injured person.

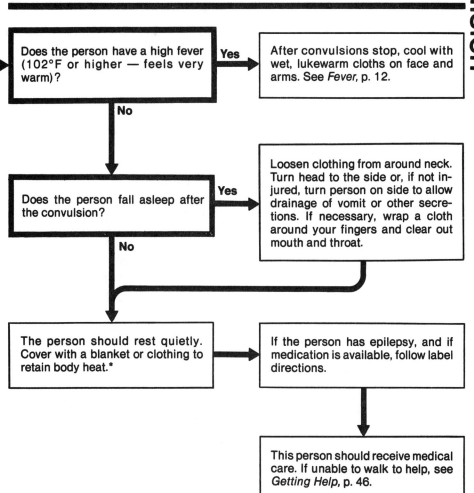

Does the person have a high fever (102°F or higher — feels very warm)?

Yes → After convulsions stop, cool with wet, lukewarm cloths on face and arms. See *Fever*, p. 12.

No

Does the person fall asleep after the convulsion?

Yes → Loosen clothing from around neck. Turn head to the side or, if not injured, turn person on side to allow drainage of vomit or other secretions. If necessary, wrap a cloth around your fingers and clear out mouth and throat.

No

The person should rest quietly. Cover with a blanket or clothing to retain body heat.*

→ If the person has epilepsy, and if medication is available, follow label directions.

→ This person should receive medical care. If unable to walk to help, see *Getting Help*, p. 46.

*If weather is very warm and person's skin does not feel cool and clammy, covering will not be necessary.

11 Diabetic Emergencies

Signs & Symptoms
diabetic coma (early warning): flushed face/
dry skin/fruity breath odor/headache/thirst/
drowsiness/nausea/rapid pulse/possible abdominal pain or vomiting
insulin shock (early warning): hunger/weak-
ness/shakiness/faintness/heavy sweating/blurred
vision/rapid pulse/cool and clammy skin/anxiety,
restlessness, and confusion

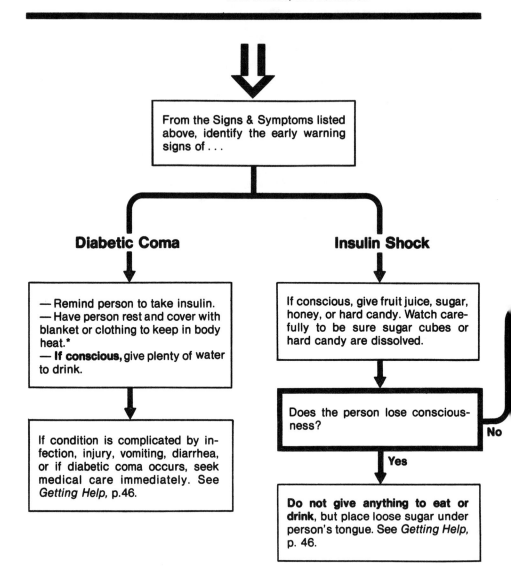

From the Signs & Symptoms listed above, identify the early warning signs of . . .

Diabetic Coma

— Remind person to take insulin.
— Have person rest and cover with blanket or clothing to keep in body heat.*
— **If conscious,** give plenty of water to drink.

If condition is complicated by infection, injury, vomiting, diarrhea, or if diabetic coma occurs, seek medical care immediately. See *Getting Help,* p.46.

Insulin Shock

If conscious, give fruit juice, sugar, honey, or hard candy. Watch carefully to be sure sugar cubes or hard candy are dissolved.

Does the person lose consciousness?

No

Yes

Do not give anything to eat or drink, but place loose sugar under person's tongue. See *Getting Help,* p. 46.

Calm the person by talking while attending to the problem. Explain what you are doing. Try not to show concern; act with confidence. Your calm behavior can help to reassure the sick person.

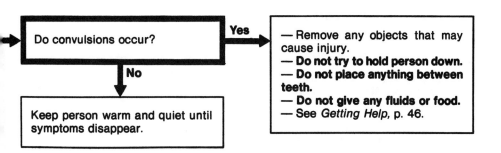

Do convulsions occur?

Yes → — Remove any objects that may cause injury.
— **Do not try to hold person down.**
— **Do not place anything between teeth.**
— **Do not give any fluids or food.**
— See *Getting Help*, p. 46.

No ↓

Keep person warm and quiet until symptoms disappear.

*If weather is very warm and person's skin does not feel cool and clammy, covering will not be necessary.

12 Fever

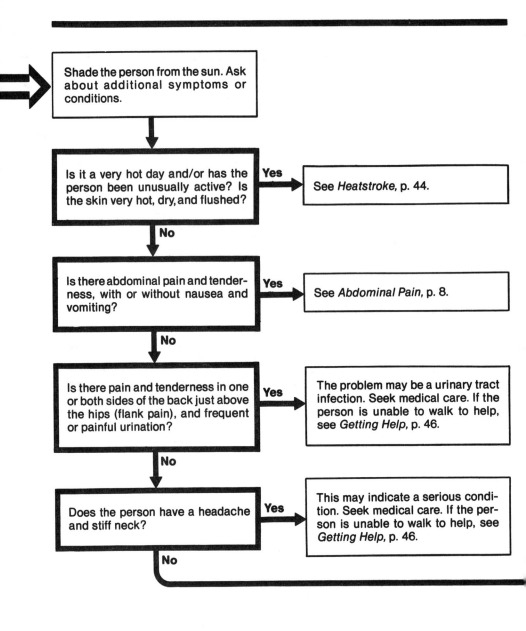

Shade the person from the sun. Ask about additional symptoms or conditions.

Is it a very hot day and/or has the person been unusually active? Is the skin very hot, dry, and flushed?

Yes → See *Heatstroke,* p. 44.

No

Is there abdominal pain and tenderness, with or without nausea and vomiting?

Yes → See *Abdominal Pain,* p. 8.

No

Is there pain and tenderness in one or both sides of the back just above the hips (flank pain), and frequent or painful urination?

Yes → The problem may be a urinary tract infection. Seek medical care. If the person is unable to walk to help, see *Getting Help,* p. 46.

No

Does the person have a headache and stiff neck?

Yes → This may indicate a serious condition. Seek medical care. If the person is unable to walk to help, see *Getting Help,* p. 46.

No

Calm the person by talking while attending to the problem. Explain what you are doing. Try not to show concern; act with confidence. Your calm behavior can help to reassure the sick person.

Suspect a viral or bacterial infection, especially if the person has a sore throat, cough, muscle pain, chills, or has been in contact with someone with similar symptoms.

Have the person rest quietly. If fever is 102°F or higher (very warm to the touch), cool body temperature with lukewarm, wet cloths on face and arms. Give aspirin or acetaminophen as directed on package.

A minor viral infection may have been the cause. Further treatment and observation will probably be unnecessary.

Watch for convulsions, especially in children. If these occur, see *Convulsion,* p. 10. Watch for: rapid breathing; cold, clammy skin; weakness. If these develop, cover person with a blanket or clothing and elevate legs with a rolled blanket, sleeping bag, etc., then see *Getting Help,* p. 46.

Yes

Does the fever drop below 102°F within 6 hours?

No

Continue wet cloths and aspirin. If fever persists or additional symptoms develop, seek medical care. If the person is unable to walk to help, see *Getting Help,* p. 46.

13 Headache

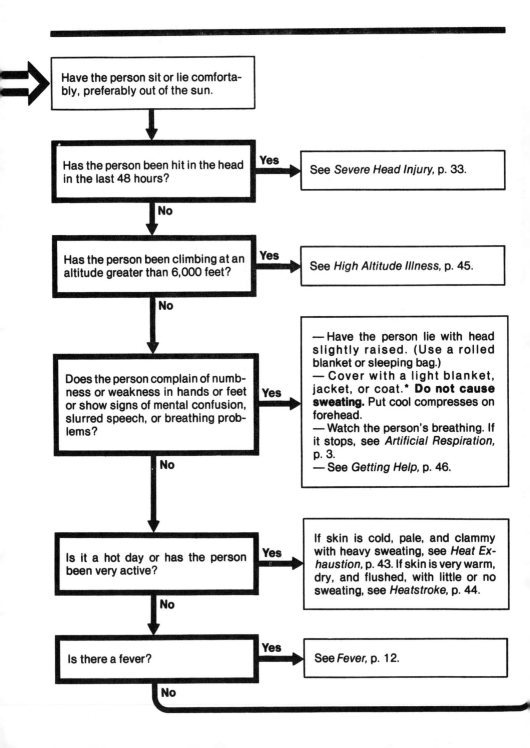

Have the person sit or lie comfortably, preferably out of the sun.

Has the person been hit in the head in the last 48 hours?

Yes → See *Severe Head Injury,* p. 33.

No

Has the person been climbing at an altitude greater than 6,000 feet?

Yes → See *High Altitude Illness,* p. 45.

No

Does the person complain of numbness or weakness in hands or feet or show signs of mental confusion, slurred speech, or breathing problems?

Yes →
— Have the person lie with head slightly raised. (Use a rolled blanket or sleeping bag.)
— Cover with a light blanket, jacket, or coat.* **Do not cause sweating.** Put cool compresses on forehead.
— Watch the person's breathing. If it stops, see *Artificial Respiration,* p. 3.
— See *Getting Help,* p. 46.

No

Is it a hot day or has the person been very active?

Yes →
If skin is cold, pale, and clammy with heavy sweating, see *Heat Exhaustion,* p. 43. If skin is very warm, dry, and flushed, with little or no sweating, see *Heatstroke,* p. 44.

No

Is there a fever?

Yes → See *Fever,* p. 12.

No

Calm the person by talking while attending to the problem. Explain what you are doing. Try not to show concern; act with confidence. Your calm behavior can help to reassure the sick or injured person.

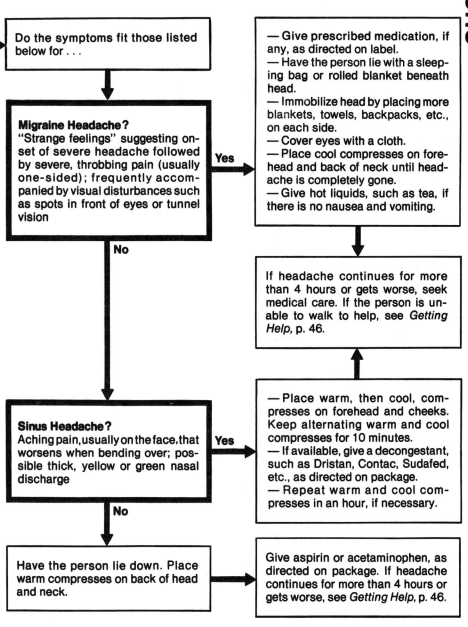

Do the symptoms fit those listed below for . . .

Migraine Headache?
"Strange feelings" suggesting onset of severe headache followed by severe, throbbing pain (usually one-sided); frequently accompanied by visual disturbances such as spots in front of eyes or tunnel vision

Yes →

— Give prescribed medication, if any, as directed on label.
— Have the person lie with a sleeping bag or rolled blanket beneath head.
— Immobilize head by placing more blankets, towels, backpacks, etc., on each side.
— Cover eyes with a cloth.
— Place cool compresses on forehead and back of neck until headache is completely gone.
— Give hot liquids, such as tea, if there is no nausea and vomiting.

If headache continues for more than 4 hours or gets worse, seek medical care. If the person is unable to walk to help, see *Getting Help,* p. 46.

No ↓

Sinus Headache?
Aching pain, usually on the face, that worsens when bending over; possible thick, yellow or green nasal discharge

Yes →

— Place warm, then cool, compresses on forehead and cheeks. Keep alternating warm and cool compresses for 10 minutes.
— If available, give a decongestant, such as Dristan, Contac, Sudafed, etc., as directed on package.
— Repeat warm and cool compresses in an hour, if necessary.

No ↓

Have the person lie down. Place warm compresses on back of head and neck.

Give aspirin or acetaminophen, as directed on package. If headache continues for more than 4 hours or gets worse, see *Getting Help,* p. 46.

*If weather is very warm and person's skin does not feel cool and clammy, covering will not be necessary.

14 Nausea & Vomiting

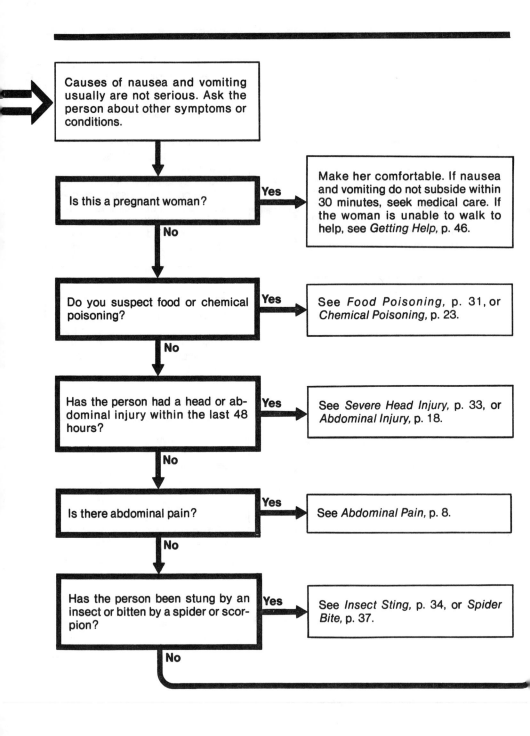

Causes of nausea and vomiting usually are not serious. Ask the person about other symptoms or conditions.

Is this a pregnant woman? **Yes** → Make her comfortable. If nausea and vomiting do not subside within 30 minutes, seek medical care. If the woman is unable to walk to help, see *Getting Help,* p. 46.

No

Do you suspect food or chemical poisoning? **Yes** → See *Food Poisoning,* p. 31, or *Chemical Poisoning,* p. 23.

No

Has the person had a head or abdominal injury within the last 48 hours? **Yes** → See *Severe Head Injury,* p. 33, or *Abdominal Injury,* p. 18.

No

Is there abdominal pain? **Yes** → See *Abdominal Pain,* p. 8.

No

Has the person been stung by an insect or bitten by a spider or scorpion? **Yes** → See *Insect Sting,* p. 34, or *Spider Bite,* p. 37.

No

Calm the person by talking while attending to the problem. Explain what you are doing. Try not to show concern; act with confidence. Your calm behavior can help to reassure the sick or injured person.

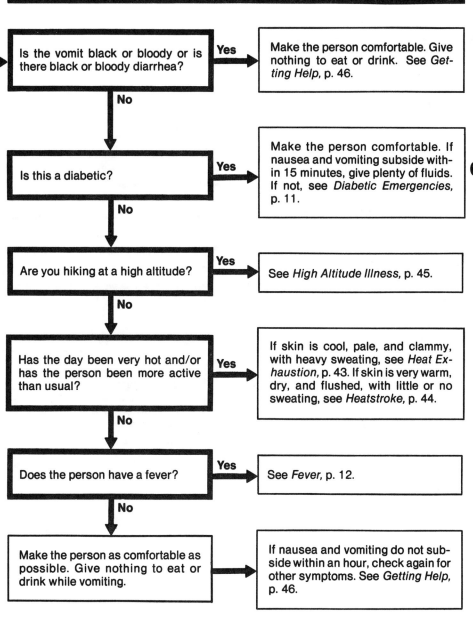

Is the vomit black or bloody or is there black or bloody diarrhea?

Yes → Make the person comfortable. Give nothing to eat or drink. See *Getting Help*, p. 46.

No

Is this a diabetic?

Yes → Make the person comfortable. If nausea and vomiting subside within 15 minutes, give plenty of fluids. If not, see *Diabetic Emergencies*, p. 11.

No

Are you hiking at a high altitude?

Yes → See *High Altitude Illness*, p. 45.

No

Has the day been very hot and/or has the person been more active than usual?

Yes → If skin is cool, pale, and clammy, with heavy sweating, see *Heat Exhaustion*, p. 43. If skin is very warm, dry, and flushed, with little or no sweating, see *Heatstroke*, p. 44.

No

Does the person have a fever?

Yes → See *Fever*, p. 12.

No

Make the person as comfortable as possible. Give nothing to eat or drink while vomiting.

→ If nausea and vomiting do not subside within an hour, check again for other symptoms. See *Getting Help*, p. 46.

15 Nosebleed

Do not stuff cotton or tissues into the nose.

If person fell or received a head injury, see *Severe Head Injury*, p. 33.

Have person sit down, leaning forward with chin toward chest.

Was person hit in nose and is there swelling?

Yes → Nose may be fractured. **Do not attempt to set the fracture.**

No

Pinch the nostrils together with thumb and forefinger. Do not squeeze hard enough to cause pain.

Apply constant pressure for 5-6 minutes. Has the bleeding stopped?

Y

No

Apply a cold, wet compress to bridge of nose. If bleeding is very heavy, keep person sitting forward and catch blood in a container to prevent choking.

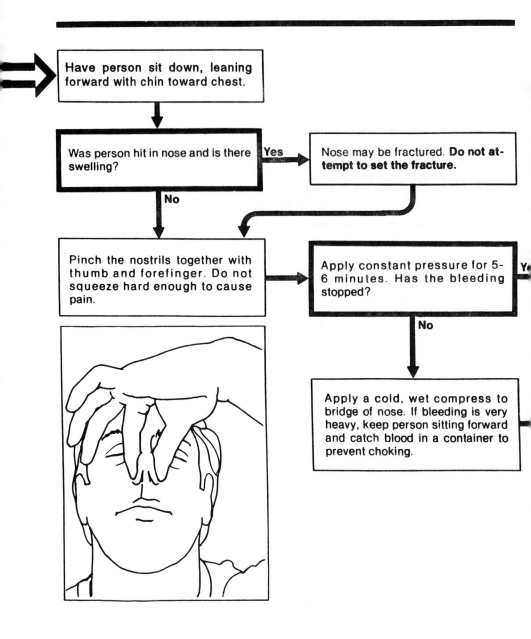

Calm the person by talking while attending to the problem. Explain what you are doing. Try not to show concern; act with confidence. Your calm behavior can help to reassure the sick or injured person.

To avoid disturbing the clot, have the person refrain from blowing nose, moving or touching the nose in any way, or talking for one hour. If you suspect a fracture, seek medical care.

Watch for: cold, clammy skin; weakness; rapid breathing. If these symptoms develop, have person lie with head raised on rolled sleeping bag, blanket, etc. Cover with a blanket or clothing to keep in body heat.

If bleeding is still uncontrolled or if you suspect a fracture, seek medical care. If person is unable to walk, see *Getting Help,* p. 46.

16 Toothache or Lost or Broken Tooth

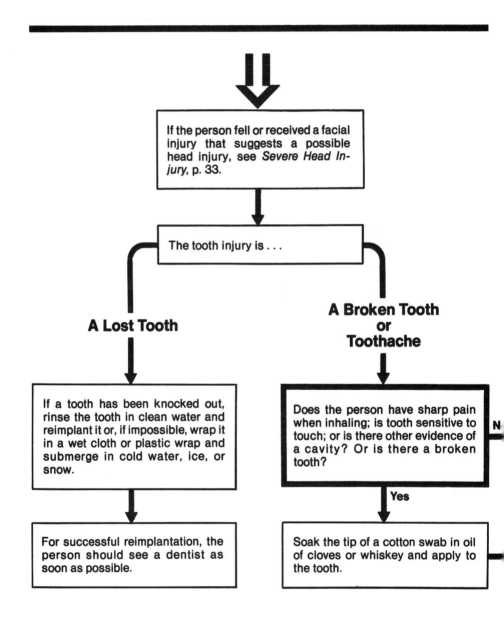

If the person fell or received a facial injury that suggests a possible head injury, see *Severe Head Injury,* p. 33.

The tooth injury is . . .

A Lost Tooth

A Broken Tooth or Toothache

If a tooth has been knocked out, rinse the tooth in clean water and reimplant it or, if impossible, wrap it in a wet cloth or plastic wrap and submerge in cold water, ice, or snow.

Does the person have sharp pain when inhaling; is tooth sensitive to touch; or is there other evidence of a cavity? Or is there a broken tooth?

N

Yes

For successful reimplantation, the person should see a dentist as soon as possible.

Soak the tip of a cotton swab in oil of cloves or whiskey and apply to the tooth.

Calm the person by talking while attending to the problem. Explain what you are doing. Try not to show concern; act with confidence. Your calm behavior can help to reassure the injured person.

Apply hot packs to the side of face to lessen pain.

Melt or rub between your palms a piece of paraffin or candle; mix in some strands of cotton. When wax mixture begins to cool, apply to the tooth as a temporary filling.

Give aspirin or acetaminophen tablets for pain. Follow label directions.

Have the person rest in a comfortable position. Lying flat may increase pain, so use rolled blankets, towels, or sleeping bag behind head and shoulders.

Person should see a dentist as soon as possible to avoid the possibility of infection developing or progressing.

17 Unconsciousness
(Lasting more than a few minutes)

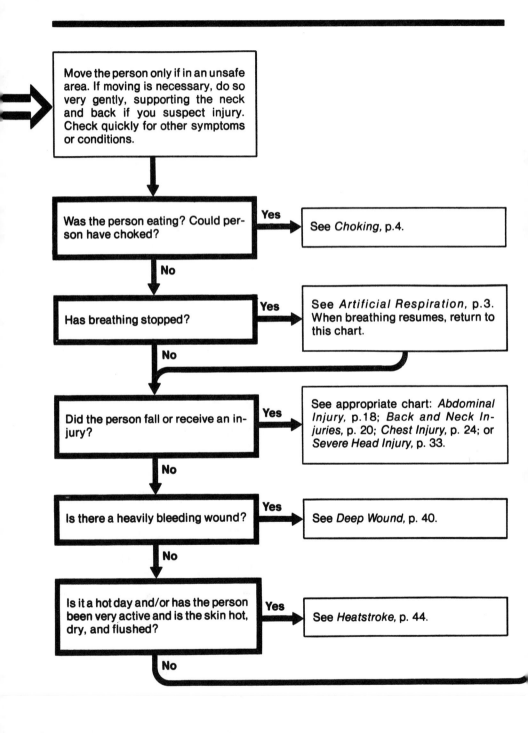

Move the person only if in an unsafe area. If moving is necessary, do so very gently, supporting the neck and back if you suspect injury. Check quickly for other symptoms or conditions.

Was the person eating? Could person have choked?

Yes → See *Choking*, p.4.

No

Has breathing stopped?

Yes → See *Artificial Respiration*, p.3. When breathing resumes, return to this chart.

No

Did the person fall or receive an injury?

Yes → See appropriate chart: *Abdominal Injury*, p.18; *Back and Neck Injuries*, p. 20; *Chest Injury*, p. 24; or *Severe Head Injury*, p. 33.

No

Is there a heavily bleeding wound?

Yes → See *Deep Wound*, p. 40.

No

Is it a hot day and/or has the person been very active and is the skin hot, dry, and flushed?

Yes → See *Heatstroke*, p. 44.

No

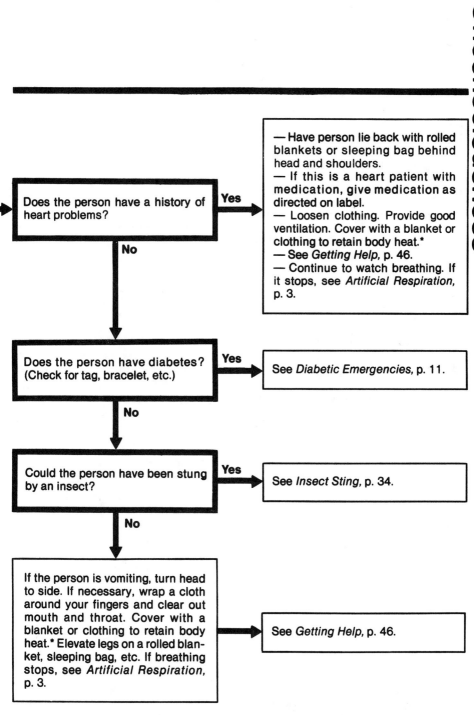

Does the person have a history of heart problems?

Yes

— Have person lie back with rolled blankets or sleeping bag behind head and shoulders.
— If this is a heart patient with medication, give medication as directed on label.
— Loosen clothing. Provide good ventilation. Cover with a blanket or clothing to retain body heat.*
— See *Getting Help,* p. 46.
— Continue to watch breathing. If it stops, see *Artificial Respiration,* p. 3.

No

Does the person have diabetes? (Check for tag, bracelet, etc.)

Yes

See *Diabetic Emergencies,* p. 11.

No

Could the person have been stung by an insect?

Yes

See *Insect Sting,* p. 34.

No

If the person is vomiting, turn head to side. If necessary, wrap a cloth around your fingers and clear out mouth and throat. Cover with a blanket or clothing to retain body heat.* Elevate legs on a rolled blanket, sleeping bag, etc. If breathing stops, see *Artificial Respiration,* p. 3.

See *Getting Help,* p. 46.

*If weather is very warm and person's skin does not feel cool and clammy, covering will not be necessary.

18 Abdominal Injury

Signs & Symptoms
Internal bleeding: swelling, discoloration, and/or severe pain/cold, clammy skin/restlessness/ thirst/vomiting or coughing blood/blood in urine or feces
Hernia: pain, swelling, or discoloration in groin or scrotum

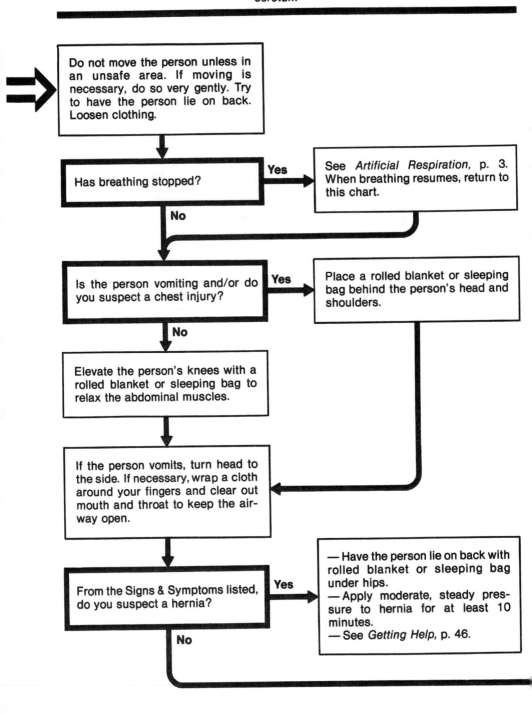

Do not move the person unless in an unsafe area. If moving is necessary, do so very gently. Try to have the person lie on back. Loosen clothing.

Has breathing stopped? — **Yes** → See *Artificial Respiration,* p. 3. When breathing resumes, return to this chart.

No

Is the person vomiting and/or do you suspect a chest injury? — **Yes** → Place a rolled blanket or sleeping bag behind the person's head and shoulders.

No

Elevate the person's knees with a rolled blanket or sleeping bag to relax the abdominal muscles.

If the person vomits, turn head to the side. If necessary, wrap a cloth around your fingers and clear out mouth and throat to keep the airway open.

From the Signs & Symptoms listed, do you suspect a hernia? — **Yes** → — Have the person lie on back with rolled blanket or sleeping bag under hips.
— Apply moderate, steady pressure to hernia for at least 10 minutes.
— See *Getting Help,* p. 46.

No

Calm the person by talking while attending to the problem. Explain what you are doing. Try not to show concern; act with confidence. Your calm behavior can help to reassure the injured person.

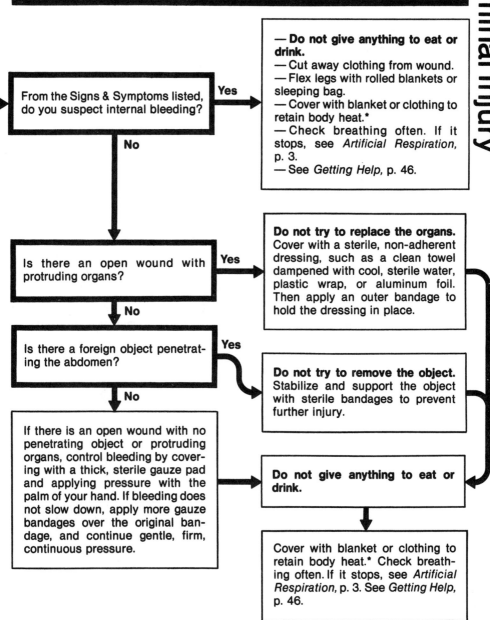

From the Signs & Symptoms listed, do you suspect internal bleeding?

Yes →

— **Do not give anything to eat or drink.**
— Cut away clothing from wound.
— Flex legs with rolled blankets or sleeping bag.
— Cover with blanket or clothing to retain body heat.*
— Check breathing often. If it stops, see *Artificial Respiration,* p. 3.
— See *Getting Help,* p. 46.

No ↓

Is there an open wound with protruding organs?

Yes →

Do not try to replace the organs. Cover with a sterile, non-adherent dressing, such as a clean towel dampened with cool, sterile water, plastic wrap, or aluminum foil. Then apply an outer bandage to hold the dressing in place.

No ↓

Is there a foreign object penetrating the abdomen?

Yes →

Do not try to remove the object. Stabilize and support the object with sterile bandages to prevent further injury.

No ↓

If there is an open wound with no penetrating object or protruding organs, control bleeding by covering with a thick, sterile gauze pad and applying pressure with the palm of your hand. If bleeding does not slow down, apply more gauze bandages over the original bandage, and continue gentle, firm, continuous pressure.

→ **Do not give anything to eat or drink.**

↓

Cover with blanket or clothing to retain body heat.* Check breathing often. If it stops, see *Artificial Respiration,* p. 3. See *Getting Help,* p. 46.

*If weather is very warm and person's skin does not feel cool and clammy, covering will not be necessary.

19 Animal Bites

In the case of an animal bite, the animal needs to be captured for observation to check for rabies. Do not attempt to do this yourself. Contact the EMS, police and animal control center. Tell them what the animal looked like and where it was seen.

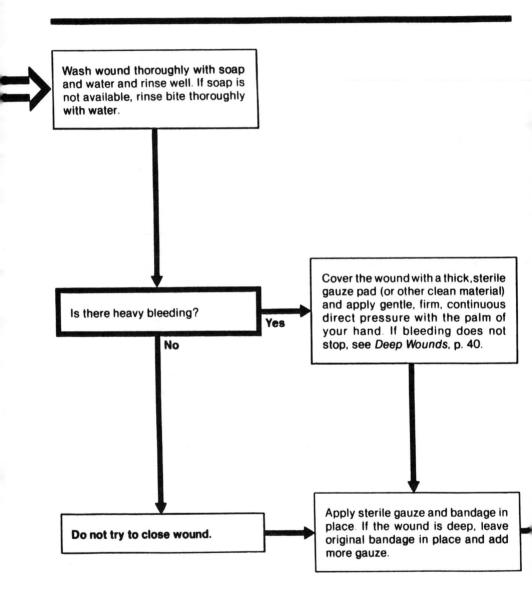

Wash wound thoroughly with soap and water and rinse well. If soap is not available, rinse bite thoroughly with water.

Is there heavy bleeding?

No

Yes

Cover the wound with a thick, sterile gauze pad (or other clean material) and apply gentle, firm, continuous direct pressure with the palm of your hand. If bleeding does not stop, see *Deep Wounds*, p. 40.

Do not try to close wound.

Apply sterile gauze and bandage in place. If the wound is deep, leave original bandage in place and add more gauze.

Calm the person by talking while attending to the problem. Explain what you are doing. Try not to show concern; act with confidence. Your calm behavior can help to reassure the injured person.

When bleeding stops, remove bandage to allow drainage — unless wound is likely to become dirty.

If the wounds are severe, check breathing. If it stops, see *Artificial Respiration,* p.3.

Watch for: cold, clammy skin; weakness; rapid breathing. If these develop, cover with a blanket or clothing to keep in body heat. If no heart problems or head injuries are present, elevate the legs on a rolled blanket or sleeping bag.

Seek medical attention. If person is unable to walk, see *Getting Help,* p. 46.

Back & Neck Injuries

Signs & Symptoms: *Severe pain and tenderness at site of injury/possible deformity of injured area/ possible paralysis of one or more limbs/pain on movement*

Do not move someone with severe back or neck injuries unless absolutely necessary.

With any severe fall or other severe trauma injuring the back, assume fractures of both neck and back.

Secure the neck with a collar (use rolled towel, etc.). Be sure to keep the head straight; do not raise or lower chin or turn head.

Has breathing stopped? — **Yes** → If not already lying on back, gently roll the person over, keeping neck and back as straight as possible. See *Artificial Respiration*, p. 3. When breathing resumes, return to this chart.

No

Is the person lying in a safe area? — **Yes** → Leave in present position. Immobilize by placing rolled blankets, sleeping bags, clothing, etc., around the entire body. Cover with a blanket or clothing to retain body heat.* See *Getting Help*, p. 46.

No

Are there 2 or more rescuers? — **Yes** → Move as shown, supporting head, limbs, and body. Cover with a blanket or clothing to retain body heat.* See *Getting Help*, p. 46.

No

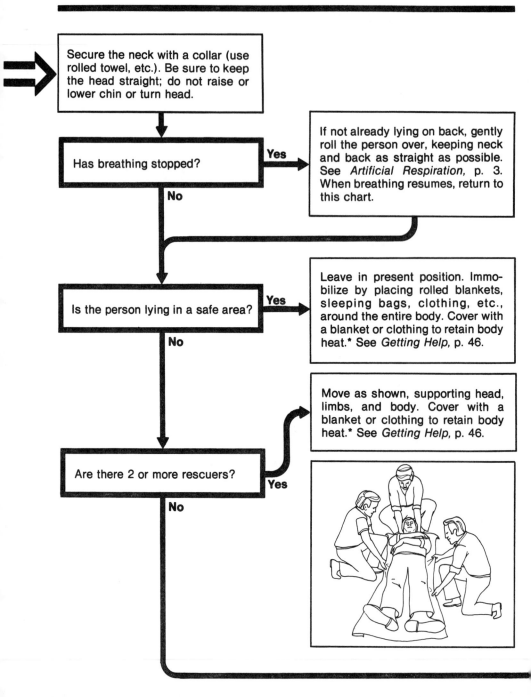

Calm the person by talking while attending to the problem. Explain what you are doing. Try not to show concern; act with confidence. Your calm behavior can help to reassure the injured person.

Leave the person in present position. Try to gently turn person onto a ground sheet or sleeping bag without bending neck or back.

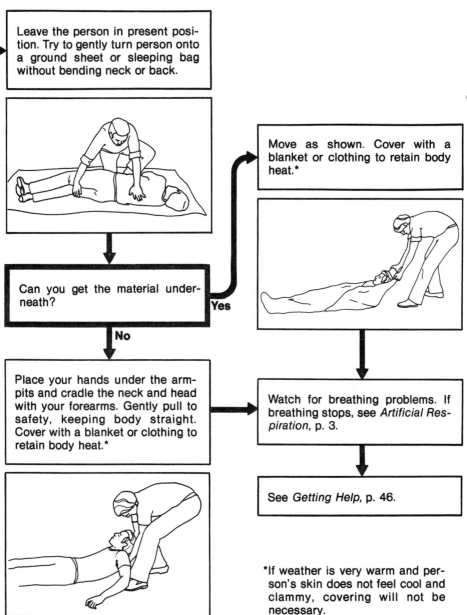

Can you get the material underneath?

Yes

Move as shown. Cover with a blanket or clothing to retain body heat.*

No

Place your hands under the armpits and cradle the neck and head with your forearms. Gently pull to safety, keeping body straight. Cover with a blanket or clothing to retain body heat.*

Watch for breathing problems. If breathing stops, see *Artificial Respiration*, p. 3.

See *Getting Help*, p. 46.

*If weather is very warm and person's skin does not feel cool and clammy, covering will not be necessary.

21 Bruise

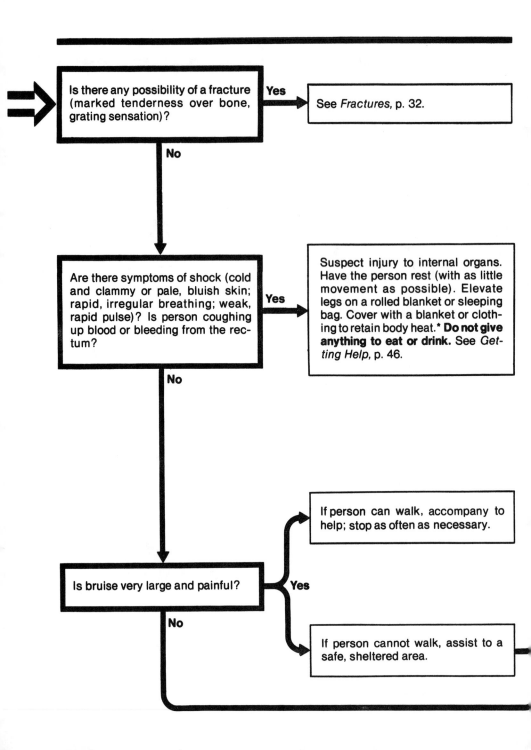

Is there any possibility of a fracture (marked tenderness over bone, grating sensation)?

Yes → See *Fractures*, p. 32.

No

Are there symptoms of shock (cold and clammy or pale, bluish skin; rapid, irregular breathing; weak, rapid pulse)? Is person coughing up blood or bleeding from the rectum?

Yes → Suspect injury to internal organs. Have the person rest (with as little movement as possible). Elevate legs on a rolled blanket or sleeping bag. Cover with a blanket or clothing to retain body heat.* **Do not give anything to eat or drink.** See *Getting Help*, p. 46.

No

Is bruise very large and painful?

Yes →

If person can walk, accompany to help; stop as often as necessary.

If person cannot walk, assist to a safe, sheltered area.

No

Calm the person by talking while attending to the problem. Explain what you are doing. Try not to show concern; act with confidence. Your calm behavior can help to reassure the injured person.

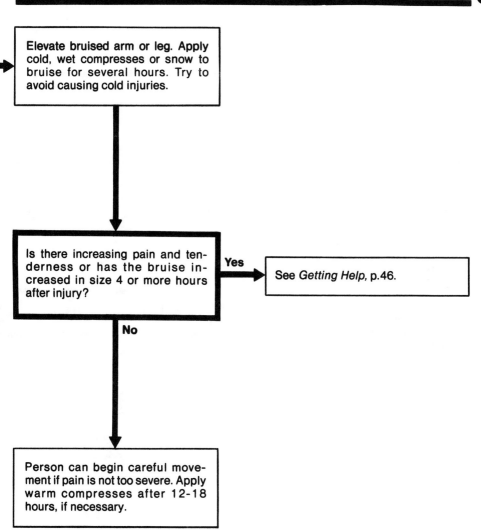

Elevate bruised arm or leg. Apply cold, wet compresses or snow to bruise for several hours. Try to avoid causing cold injuries.

Is there increasing pain and tenderness or has the bruise increased in size 4 or more hours after injury?

Yes See *Getting Help,* p.46.

No

Person can begin careful movement if pain is not too severe. Apply warm compresses after 12-18 hours, if necessary.

*If weather is very warm and person's skin does not feel cool and clammy, covering will not be necessary.

22 Burns

(Including Lightning, Chemical Burns, and Sunburn)

First Degree: *redness of skin/pain, perhaps with mild swelling. First degree burns involving over 10% of the body should be considered third degree.*
Second Degree: *deep reddening of skin/skin has glossy appearance from leaking fluid (plasma)/ possible loss of some skin/blisters. Second degree burns involving over 10% of the body should be considered third degree.*
Third Degree: *loss of all skin layers/possible charring of skin edges involving more than a very small area*

If the person was struck by lightning, check neck artery for pulse. If no pulse, see *CPR*, p. 5. When heartbeat resumes, return to this page.

Gently move the person to a safe, sheltered area. Remove clothing from the burn area (cut away if necessary). If some clothing sticks to the burn, do not try to remove it.

First Degree

Second Degree

Apply cold, wet compresses to burned area, or immerse burn in fresh, cold water — not ice or salt water.

No ← Are there open blisters?

Continue cold water applications until pain subsides (usually about 15-20 minutes). Apply loose, moist, sterile dressing and bandage.

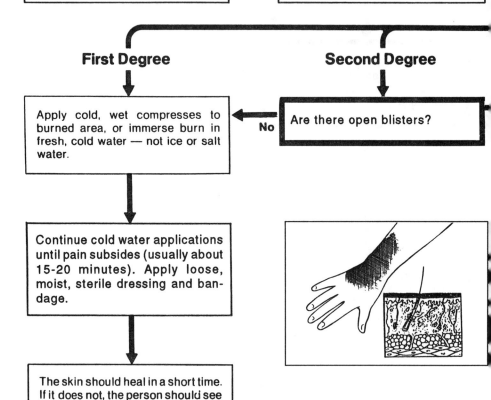

The skin should heal in a short time. If it does not, the person should see a doctor.

Calm the person by talking while attending to the problem. Explain what you are doing. Try not to show concern; act with confidence. Your calm behavior can help to reassure the injured person.

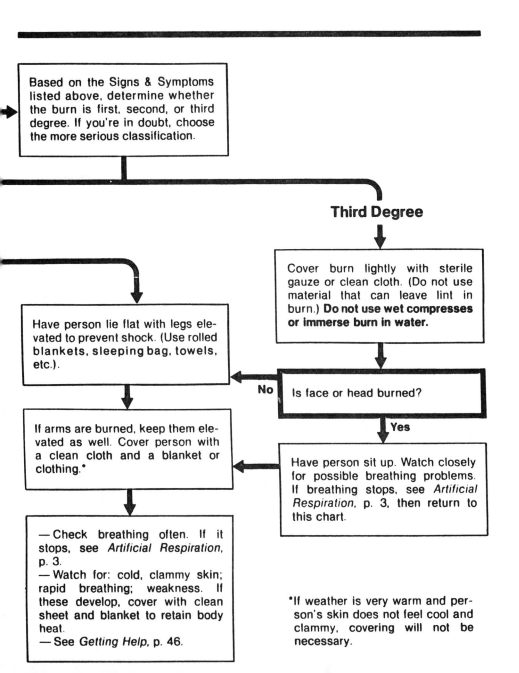

Based on the Signs & Symptoms listed above, determine whether the burn is first, second, or third degree. If you're in doubt, choose the more serious classification.

Third Degree

Cover burn lightly with sterile gauze or clean cloth. (Do not use material that can leave lint in burn.) **Do not use wet compresses or immerse burn in water.**

Have person lie flat with legs elevated to prevent shock. (Use rolled blankets, sleeping bag, towels, etc.).

No ← Is face or head burned?

Yes

If arms are burned, keep them elevated as well. Cover person with a clean cloth and a blanket or clothing.*

Have person sit up. Watch closely for possible breathing problems. If breathing stops, see *Artificial Respiration*, p. 3, then return to this chart.

—Check breathing often. If it stops, see *Artificial Respiration*, p. 3.
—Watch for: cold, clammy skin; rapid breathing; weakness. If these develop, cover with clean sheet and blanket to retain body heat.
—See *Getting Help*, p. 46.

*If weather is very warm and person's skin does not feel cool and clammy, covering will not be necessary.

23 Chemical Poisoning

Signs & Symptoms: *an empty container of known poison/sudden onset of abdominal or generalized pain/nausea and vomiting may or may not be present/burns on lips and mouth/distinctive breath odor/stupor or unconsciousness. Symptoms will vary depending on type of poison.*

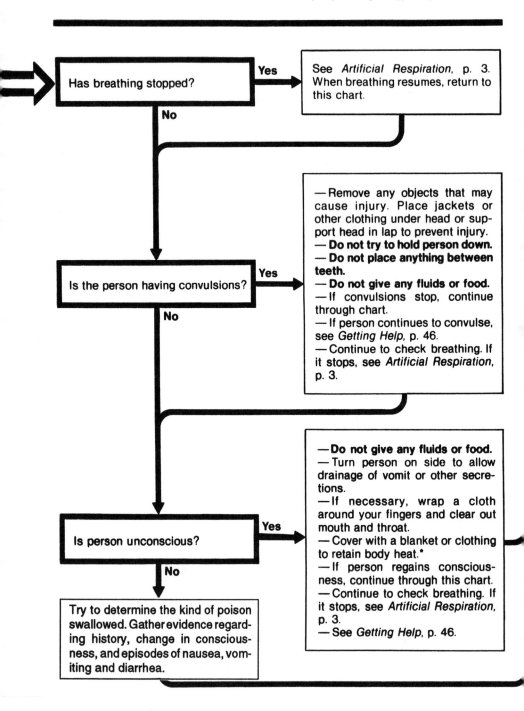

Has breathing stopped? — **Yes** → See *Artificial Respiration*, p. 3. When breathing resumes, return to this chart.

No

Is the person having convulsions? — **Yes** →
—Remove any objects that may cause injury. Place jackets or other clothing under head or support head in lap to prevent injury.
— **Do not try to hold person down.**
— **Do not place anything between teeth.**
— **Do not give any fluids or food.**
—If convulsions stop, continue through chart.
—If person continues to convulse, see *Getting Help*, p. 46.
—Continue to check breathing. If it stops, see *Artificial Respiration*, p. 3.

No

Is person unconscious? — **Yes** →
— **Do not give any fluids or food.**
— Turn person on side to allow drainage of vomit or other secretions.
—If necessary, wrap a cloth around your fingers and clear out mouth and throat.
— Cover with a blanket or clothing to retain body heat.*
—If person regains consciousness, continue through this chart.
—Continue to check breathing. If it stops, see *Artificial Respiration*, p. 3.
— See *Getting Help*, p. 46.

No

Try to determine the kind of poison swallowed. Gather evidence regarding history, change in consciousness, and episodes of nausea, vomiting and diarrhea.

Calm the person by talking while attending to the problem. Explain what you are doing. Try not to show concern; act with confidence. Your calm behavior can help to reassure the sick person.

Are there clues that suggest a strong corrosive poison or petroleum product:
— burns on the lips and mouth?
— breath odor of gasoline, kerosene, or turpentine?
— information on bottle or can label?

Yes

— **Do not induce vomiting.**
— Dilute by giving a bottle of milk or water.

No

Try to induce vomiting by giving the person the following:
— 2 tbsp. syrup of ipecac with 1-2 glasses of water (adult)
— 1 tbsp. syrup of ipecac with 1-2 glasses of water (<10 yrs.)
If they haven't vomited in 20 minutes, repeat the dose.

Without syrup of ipecac, vomiting can be induced with the "gag" reflex. Lean the victim forward, reach into the mouth with a couple of fingers and tickle the back of the throat.

Keep person calm and warm. Have the person sit up with rolled blankets or sleeping bag behind head and shoulders.

Continue to watch for breathing problems. If these develop, see *Artificial Respiration*, p. 3.

Seek medical care. See *Getting Help*, p. 46.

*If weather is very warm and person's skin does not feel cool and clammy, covering will not be necessary.

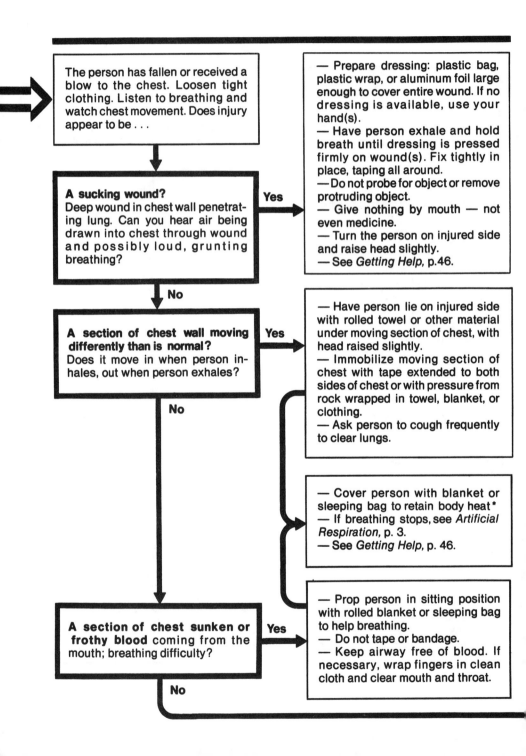

The person has fallen or received a blow to the chest. Loosen tight clothing. Listen to breathing and watch chest movement. Does injury appear to be . . .

A sucking wound?
Deep wound in chest wall penetrating lung. Can you hear air being drawn into chest through wound and possibly loud, grunting breathing?

Yes →
— Prepare dressing: plastic bag, plastic wrap, or aluminum foil large enough to cover entire wound. If no dressing is available, use your hand(s).
— Have person exhale and hold breath until dressing is pressed firmly on wound(s). Fix tightly in place, taping all around.
— Do not probe for object or remove protruding object.
— Give nothing by mouth — not even medicine.
— Turn the person on injured side and raise head slightly.
— See *Getting Help*, p.46.

No

A section of chest wall moving differently than is normal?
Does it move in when person inhales, out when person exhales?

Yes →
— Have person lie on injured side with rolled towel or other material under moving section of chest, with head raised slightly.
— Immobilize moving section of chest with tape extended to both sides of chest or with pressure from rock wrapped in towel, blanket, or clothing.
— Ask person to cough frequently to clear lungs.

No

— Cover person with blanket or sleeping bag to retain body heat*
— If breathing stops, see *Artificial Respiration*, p. 3.
— See *Getting Help*, p. 46.

A section of chest sunken or frothy blood coming from the mouth; breathing difficulty?

Yes →
— Prop person in sitting position with rolled blanket or sleeping bag to help breathing.
— Do not tape or bandage.
— Keep airway free of blood. If necessary, wrap fingers in clean cloth and clear mouth and throat.

No

Calm the person by talking while attending to the problem. Explain what you are doing. Try not to show concern; act with confidence. Your calm behavior can help to reassure the injured person.

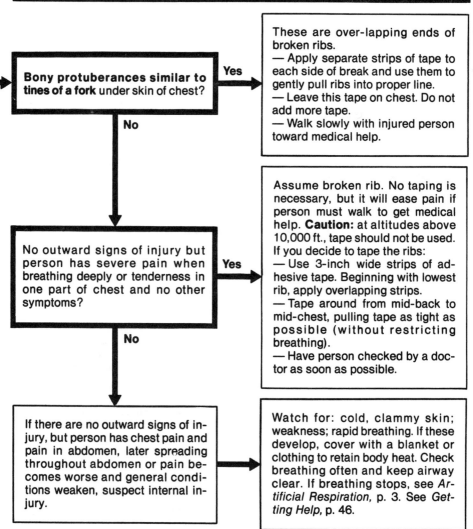

Bony protuberances similar to tines of a fork under skin of chest?

Yes

These are over-lapping ends of broken ribs.
— Apply separate strips of tape to each side of break and use them to gently pull ribs into proper line.
— Leave this tape on chest. Do not add more tape.
— Walk slowly with injured person toward medical help.

No

No outward signs of injury but person has severe pain when breathing deeply or tenderness in one part of chest and no other symptoms?

Yes

Assume broken rib. No taping is necessary, but it will ease pain if person must walk to get medical help. **Caution:** at altitudes above 10,000 ft., tape should not be used. If you decide to tape the ribs:
— Use 3-inch wide strips of adhesive tape. Beginning with lowest rib, apply overlapping strips.
— Tape around from mid-back to mid-chest, pulling tape as tight as possible (without restricting breathing).
— Have person checked by a doctor as soon as possible.

No

If there are no outward signs of injury, but person has chest pain and pain in abdomen, later spreading throughout abdomen or pain becomes worse and general conditions weaken, suspect internal injury.

Watch for: cold, clammy skin; weakness; rapid breathing. If these develop, cover with a blanket or clothing to retain body heat. Check breathing often and keep airway clear. If breathing stops, see *Artificial Respiration*, p. 3. See *Getting Help*, p. 46.

*If weather is very warm and person's skin does not feel cool and clammy, covering will not be necessary.

25 Minor Cuts
(Including Rope Burns)

Definition: *minor bleeding/no involvement of underlying tissue (muscle, nerve, tendon)*

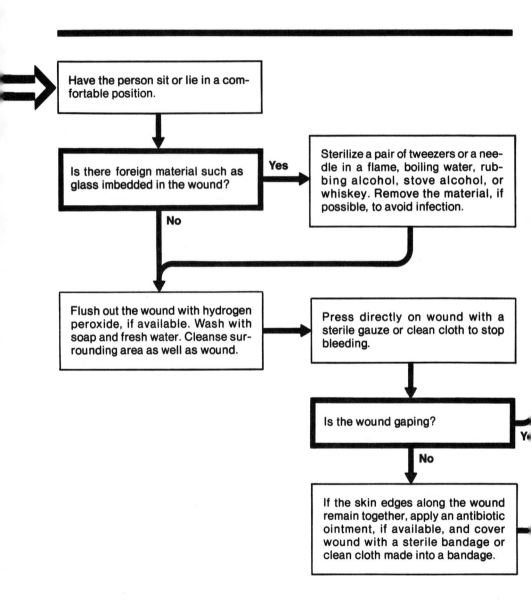

Have the person sit or lie in a comfortable position.

Is there foreign material such as glass imbedded in the wound?

Yes → Sterilize a pair of tweezers or a needle in a flame, boiling water, rubbing alcohol, stove alcohol, or whiskey. Remove the material, if possible, to avoid infection.

No

Flush out the wound with hydrogen peroxide, if available. Wash with soap and fresh water. Cleanse surrounding area as well as wound.

Press directly on wound with a sterile gauze or clean cloth to stop bleeding.

Is the wound gaping?

Y

No

If the skin edges along the wound remain together, apply an antibiotic ointment, if available, and cover wound with a sterile bandage or clean cloth made into a bandage.

Calm the person by talking while attending to the problem. Explain what you are doing. Try not to show concern; act with confidence. Your calm behavior can help to reassure the injured person.

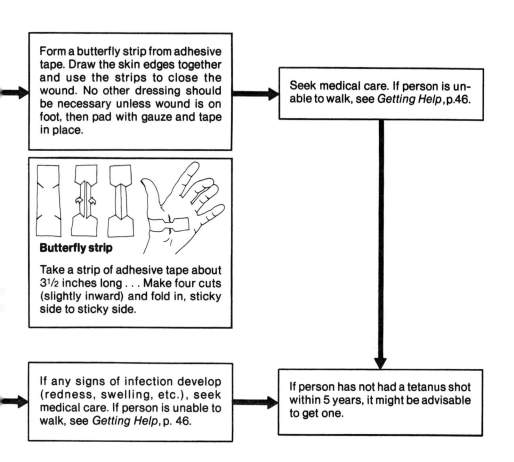

Form a butterfly strip from adhesive tape. Draw the skin edges together and use the strips to close the wound. No other dressing should be necessary unless wound is on foot, then pad with gauze and tape in place.

Butterfly strip

Take a strip of adhesive tape about 3½ inches long . . . Make four cuts (slightly inward) and fold in, sticky side to sticky side.

Seek medical care. If person is unable to walk, see *Getting Help*, p.46.

If any signs of infection develop (redness, swelling, etc.), seek medical care. If person is unable to walk, see *Getting Help*, p. 46.

If person has not had a tetanus shot within 5 years, it might be advisable to get one.

26 Dislocations

Signs & Symptoms: *distortion in shape of joint/ swelling and discoloration/pain with movement/ affected limb looks longer or shorter/loss of movement in joint.*
If you suspect Back or Neck Injury, see p. 20.

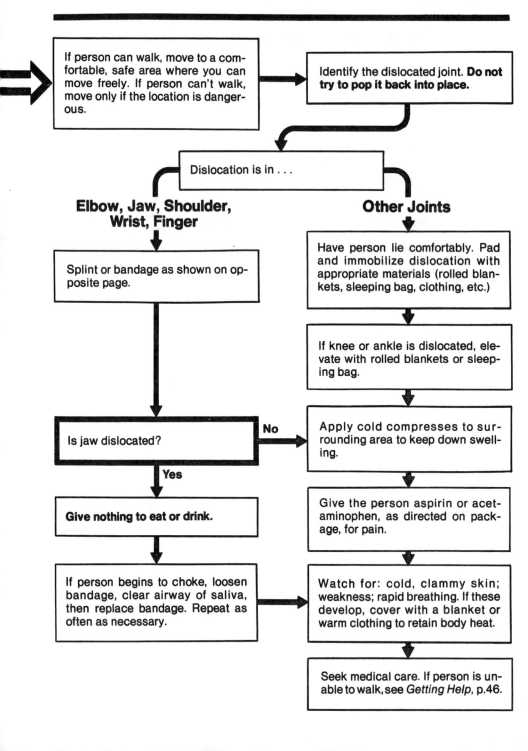

If person can walk, move to a comfortable, safe area where you can move freely. If person can't walk, move only if the location is dangerous.

Identify the dislocated joint. **Do not try to pop it back into place.**

Dislocation is in . . .

Elbow, Jaw, Shoulder, Wrist, Finger

Other Joints

Splint or bandage as shown on opposite page.

Have person lie comfortably. Pad and immobilize dislocation with appropriate materials (rolled blankets, sleeping bag, clothing, etc.)

If knee or ankle is dislocated, elevate with rolled blankets or sleeping bag.

Is jaw dislocated?

No

Apply cold compresses to surrounding area to keep down swelling.

Yes

Give nothing to eat or drink.

Give the person aspirin or acetaminophen, as directed on package, for pain.

If person begins to choke, loosen bandage, clear airway of saliva, then replace bandage. Repeat as often as necessary.

Watch for: cold, clammy skin; weakness; rapid breathing. If these develop, cover with a blanket or warm clothing to retain body heat.

Seek medical care. If person is unable to walk, see *Getting Help*, p.46.

Calm the person by talking while attending to the problem. Explain what you are doing. Try not to show concern; act with confidence. Your calm behavior can help to reassure the injured person.

Jaw

Use four-tailed bandage or two bandages crossed and tied at top and back of head.

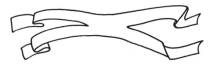

suggested materials:

4 lengths of 40" long tape
strips of cloth (bandana, large handkerchief, etc.)

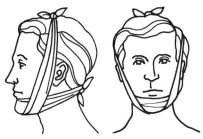

Tie over head and behind neck.

Finger

splints: closed knife, eating spoon, padded stick, other finger.

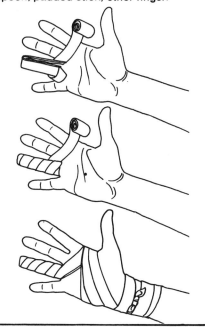

Elbow, Shoulder, or Wrist Sling

suggested materials:
shirt or jacket
large handkerchief, bandana, or piece of ground sheet folded diagonally

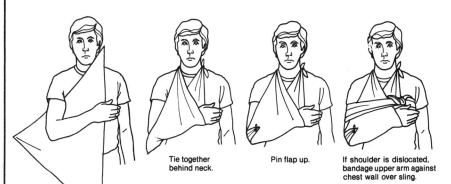

Tie together behind neck.

Pin flap up.

If shoulder is dislocated, bandage upper arm against chest wall over sling.

27 Chemical Burns of the Eyes

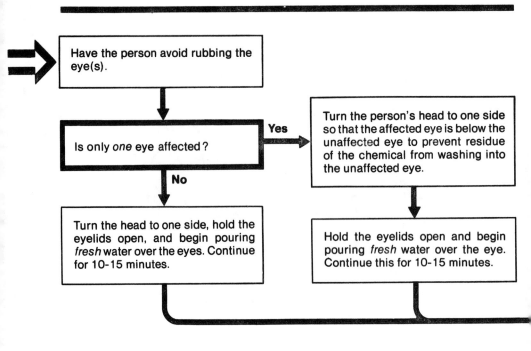

Have the person avoid rubbing the eye(s).

Is only *one* eye affected?

Yes → Turn the person's head to one side so that the affected eye is below the unaffected eye to prevent residue of the chemical from washing into the unaffected eye.

No → Turn the head to one side, hold the eyelids open, and begin pouring *fresh* water over the eyes. Continue for 10-15 minutes.

Hold the eyelids open and begin pouring *fresh* water over the eye. Continue this for 10-15 minutes.

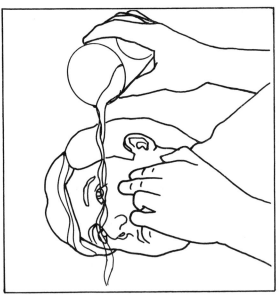

Calm the person by talking while attending to the problem. Explain what you are doing. Try not to show concern; act with confidence. Your calm behavior can help to reassure the injured person.

Remove any coagulated chemical from the eye with a clean, moistened tissue or cloth.

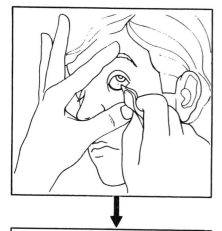

After rinsing out the eye(s) again, apply sterile gauze bandages or clean cloths to both eyes (even if only one is affected). Tie firmly in place, making sure there is no pressure against the eyes.

Seek medical care immediately. See *Getting Help*, p. 46.

28 Foreign Object in Eye
(With no injury or bleeding)

For chemicals in eye, see *Chemical Burns of the Eyes*, p. 27.

Have the person avoid rubbing the eye.

Gently open the eye and locate the object. It is under the . . .

Upper Lid

Lower Lid

Gently pull the upper lid away from the eyeball and down over the lower lid. Hold the upper lid in this position for a few seconds to allow tears to wash away the object.

Gently pull the lower lid away from the eyeball.

If object did not come out, have person look down. Clasp upper lash between thumb and forefinger and gently pull the upper lid away from the eyeball. Place a matchstick, cotton swab shaft, or other long, thin object that will not cause any injury over the lid, then turn the lid back over the stick.

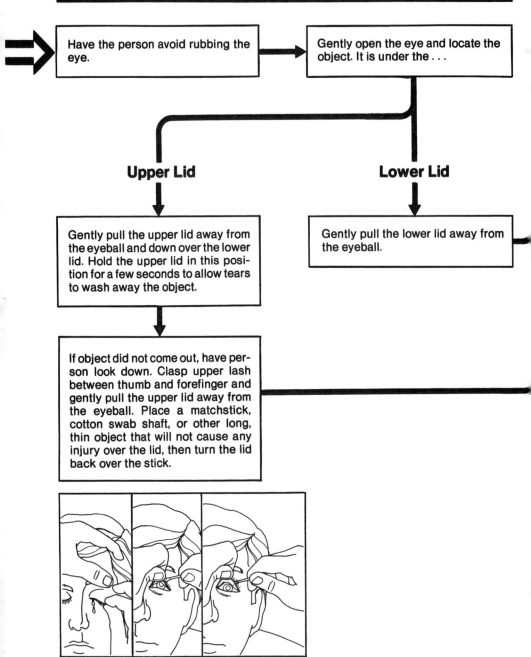

Calm the person by talking while attending to the problem. Explain what you are doing. Try not to show concern; act with confidence. Your calm behavior can help to reassure the injured person.

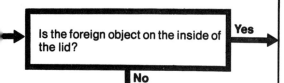

Is the foreign object on the inside of the lid?

Yes → Gently remove it with a moistened tissue or cloth or by pouring fresh water in eye. No further treatment will be necessary unless swelling, pain, or discoloration develop. If these occur, seek medical care. If person is unable to walk, see *Getting Help,* p. 46.

No ↓

If you think the object is imbedded in the cornea, do not attempt to remove it. Cover both eyes with a dry bandage. **Do not apply any pressure.** Seek medical care. See *Getting Help,* p. 46.

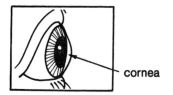

cornea

29 Eye Injury

For chemicals in the eye, see p. 27. For small foreign object in eye, but not penetrating eye, see p. 28.

Have the person lie down. Identify the type of injury.

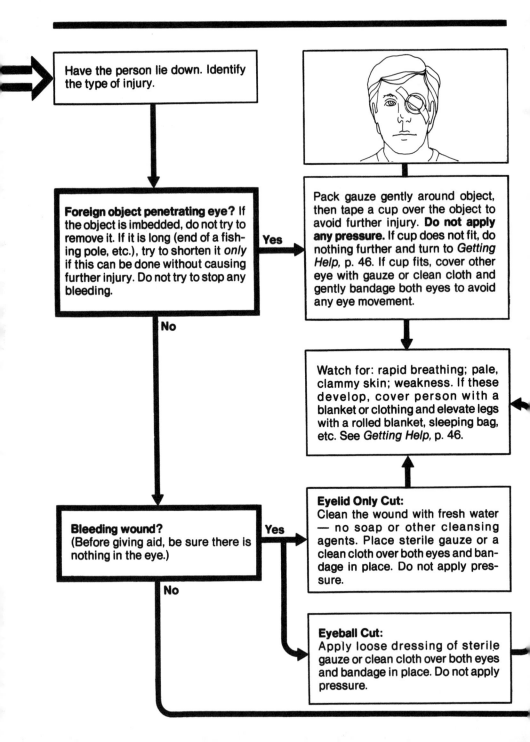

Foreign object penetrating eye? If the object is imbedded, do not try to remove it. If it is long (end of a fishing pole, etc.), try to shorten it *only* if this can be done without causing further injury. Do not try to stop any bleeding.

Yes →

Pack gauze gently around object, then tape a cup over the object to avoid further injury. **Do not apply any pressure.** If cup does not fit, do nothing further and turn to *Getting Help,* p. 46. If cup fits, cover other eye with gauze or clean cloth and gently bandage both eyes to avoid any eye movement.

No

Watch for: rapid breathing; pale, clammy skin; weakness. If these develop, cover person with a blanket or clothing and elevate legs with a rolled blanket, sleeping bag, etc. See *Getting Help,* p. 46.

Bleeding wound?
(Before giving aid, be sure there is nothing in the eye.)

Yes →

Eyelid Only Cut:
Clean the wound with fresh water — no soap or other cleansing agents. Place sterile gauze or a clean cloth over both eyes and bandage in place. Do not apply pressure.

No

Eyeball Cut:
Apply loose dressing of sterile gauze or clean cloth over both eyes and bandage in place. Do not apply pressure.

Calm the person by talking while attending to the problem. Explain what you are doing. Try not to show concern; act with confidence. Your calm behavior can help to reassure the injured person.

Severely bruised or "black" eye

Apply cold, wet compresses for 15-20 minutes to reduce swelling and discoloration.

Is pain, swelling, or discoloration extensive?

Yes → If person cannot walk to help, see *Getting Help,* p. 46.

No

The injury probably won't need any additional care, but continue to check the eye for 24 hours.

→ Does the person complain of severe pain or blurred vision, or do other symptoms develop?

Yes ↑

No

No further treatment is necessary.

30 Fishhook Removal

If the hook is imbedded in or near eyes, ears, nose, or groin, leave it in place and seek medical help immediately. If person is unable to walk, see *Getting Help,* p. 46.

No Are wire cutters, pliers, or other heavy-duty shearing devices available? **Yes**

Without Shearing Device

If barb is completely imbedded, do not attempt to remove the hook by pulling backwards.

Leave hook in place. Bandage gently to keep it from moving.

Seek medical care. If person is unable to walk, see *Getting Help,* p. 46.

With Shearing Device

Push the hook through the skin until barb is exposed.

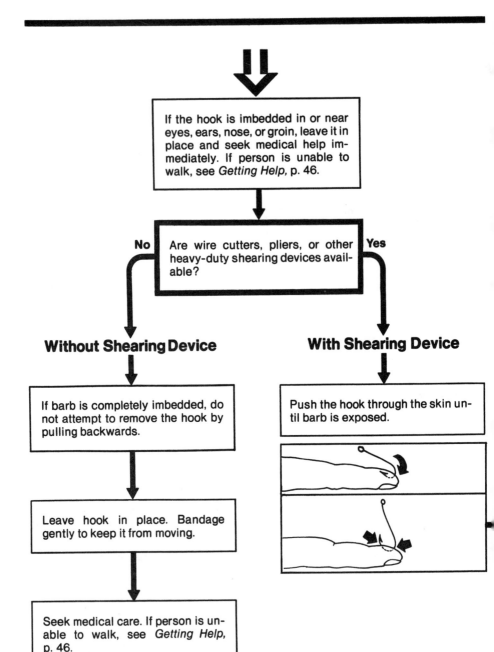

Calm the person by talking while attending to the problem. Explain what you are doing. Try not to show concern; act with confidence. Your calm behavior can help to reassure the injured person.

Cut the shank of the hook at the base of the barb. Remove the pieces.

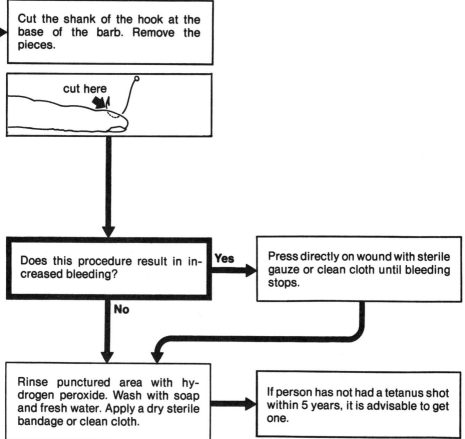

cut here

Does this procedure result in increased bleeding?

Yes → Press directly on wound with sterile gauze or clean cloth until bleeding stops.

No

Rinse punctured area with hydrogen peroxide. Wash with soap and fresh water. Apply a dry sterile bandage or clean cloth.

If person has not had a tetanus shot within 5 years, it is advisable to get one.

If the person has not vomited, induce vomiting by giving syrup of ipecac or by sticking your finger or the bowl of a spoon on back of throat.

Has the person eaten home canned or poorly stored, cooked food within last 24 hours and are the symptoms muscle weakness, headache, dizziness, slurred speech, disturbed vision, breathing difficulty, or coma?

Yes → Suspect botulism. If breathing stops, see *Artificial Respiration,* p. 3.

No

Has the person eaten shellfish within the last hour and do symptoms include numbness around face and head gradually spreading throughout entire body, dizziness, increased salivation, muscle weakness, or paralysis?

Yes → If paralysis occurs, have person drink as much baking soda solution as possible (1 tsp. to 1 glass of water).

No

If the person has eaten wild mushrooms, berries, plants, other suspicious foods or water within past 12 hours, suspect general food poisoning. Symptoms can range from nausea, vomiting, and cramps to hallucinations or slurred speech.

Calm the person by talking while attending to the problem. Explain what you are doing. Try not to show concern; act with confidence. Your calm behavior can help to reassure the sick person.

Give medicinal activated charcoal, at least 20 tablets with plenty of water. If not available, give Epsom salts.

Have person lie on side and cover with a blanket or clothing to retain body heat.*

Watch for choking and keep airway clear. If necessary, wrap cloth around fingers to clear vomit from throat. See *Getting Help*, p. 46.

*If weather is very warm and person's skin does not feel cool and clammy, covering will not be necessary.

32 Fractures

For *Severe Head Injury,* see p. 33.
For *Back or Neck Injuries,* see p. 20

Signs & Symptoms: *sound of bone snapping/ deformity with swelling and discoloration/ painful to touch/possible grating sensation of broken bone ends. With any injury, if you're not sure, assume there is a fracture.*

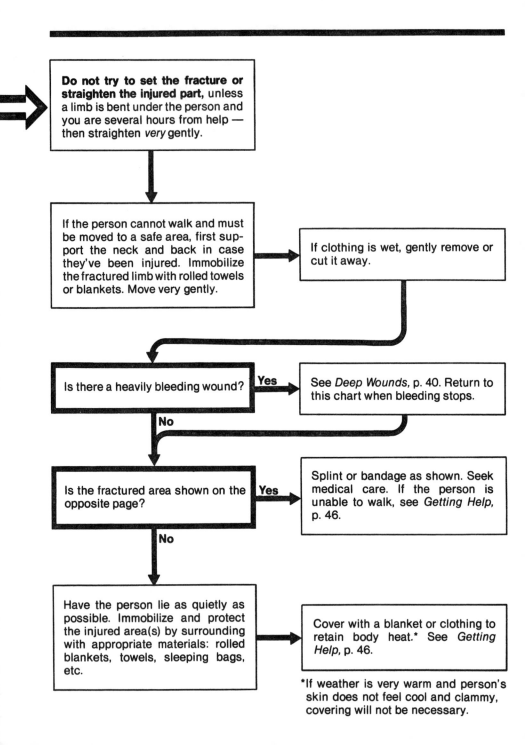

Do not try to set the fracture or straighten the injured part, unless a limb is bent under the person and you are several hours from help — then straighten *very* gently.

If the person cannot walk and must be moved to a safe area, first support the neck and back in case they've been injured. Immobilize the fractured limb with rolled towels or blankets. Move very gently.

If clothing is wet, gently remove or cut it away.

Is there a heavily bleeding wound? **Yes** → See *Deep Wounds,* p. 40. Return to this chart when bleeding stops.

No

Is the fractured area shown on the opposite page? **Yes** → Splint or bandage as shown. Seek medical care. If the person is unable to walk, see *Getting Help,* p. 46.

No

Have the person lie as quietly as possible. Immobilize and protect the injured area(s) by surrounding with appropriate materials: rolled blankets, towels, sleeping bags, etc.

Cover with a blanket or clothing to retain body heat.* See *Getting Help,* p. 46.

*If weather is very warm and person's skin does not feel cool and clammy, covering will not be necessary.

Calm the person by talking while attending to the problem. Explain what you are doing. Try not to show concern; act with confidence. Your calm behavior can help to reassure the injured person.

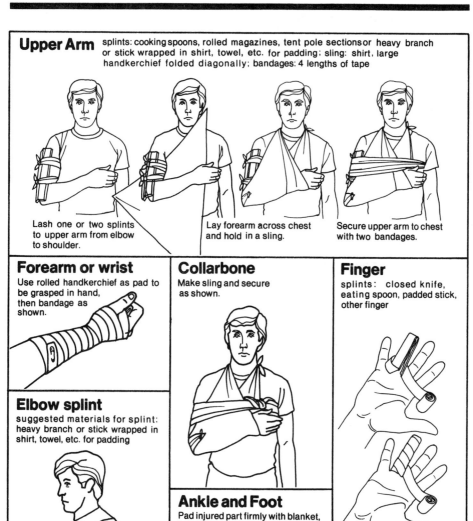

Upper Arm
splints: cooking spoons, rolled magazines, tent pole sections or heavy branch or stick wrapped in shirt, towel, etc. for padding; sling: shirt, large handkerchief folded diagonally; bandages: 4 lengths of tape

Lash one or two splints to upper arm from elbow to shoulder.

Lay forearm across chest and hold in a sling.

Secure upper arm to chest with two bandages.

Forearm or wrist
Use rolled handkerchief as pad to be grasped in hand, then bandage as shown.

Collarbone
Make sling and secure as shown.

Finger
splints: closed knife, eating spoon, padded stick, other finger

Elbow splint
suggested materials for splint: heavy branch or stick wrapped in shirt, towel, etc. for padding

Ankle and Foot
Pad injured part firmly with blanket, towels, or ground sheets. Keep leg elevated.

33 Severe Head Injury

Signs & Symptoms
Skull Fracture: *dizziness/double vision/ slurred speech/headache/possible bleeding or draining of clear fluid from ears, nose, or mouth/possible nausea and vomiting/possible convulsions/ pupils of unequal size/paralysis on the side opposite injury/deformity of the skull/One eye may appear sunken.*

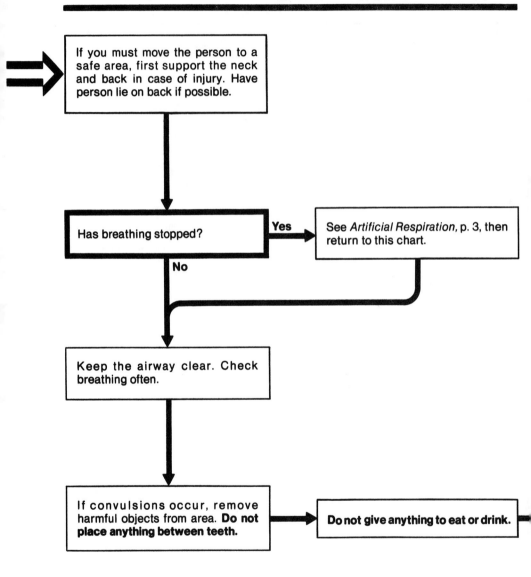

If you must move the person to a safe area, first support the neck and back in case of injury. Have person lie on back if possible.

Has breathing stopped? **Yes** → See *Artificial Respiration*, p. 3, then return to this chart.

No

Keep the airway clear. Check breathing often.

If convulsions occur, remove harmful objects from area. **Do not place anything between teeth.** → **Do not give anything to eat or drink.**

Calm the person by talking while attending to the problem. Explain what you are doing. Try not to show concern; act with confidence. Your calm behavior can help to reassure the injured person.

Is there an open wound?

Yes

Do not attempt to clean. Cover the wound with a thick, sterile gauze pad or clean cloth. Use a strip of cloth or bandage to hold pad in place. Take another strip and wrap it around the head and over the pad while pulling gently but firmly. Avoid finger pressure.

See *illustration below.*

No

Keep person quiet. Cover with a blanket or clothing to retain body heat.* If there is no neck injury, have person lie with a rolled blanket or sleeping bag beneath head and shoulders. Keep mouth clear of blood and vomit.

Continue to watch breathing. If breathing stops, see *Artificial Respiration*, p. 3.

Seek medical care immediately. See *Getting Help,* p. 46.

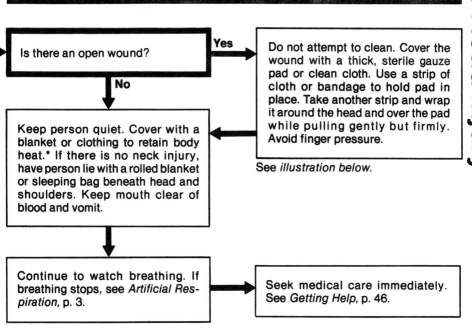

Open Wound
Direct pressure applied to wound with sterile dressing or clean cloth held in place with a head bandage.

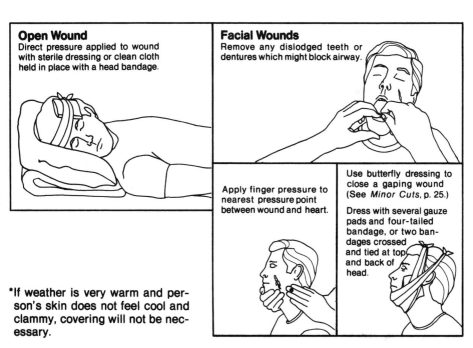

Facial Wounds
Remove any dislodged teeth or dentures which might block airway.

Apply finger pressure to nearest pressure point between wound and heart.

Use butterfly dressing to close a gaping wound (See *Minor Cuts*, p. 25.)

Dress with several gauze pads and four-tailed bandage, or two bandages crossed and tied at top and back of head.

*If weather is very warm and person's skin does not feel cool and clammy, covering will not be necessary.

34 Insect Stings

Signs & Symptoms
Emergency allergic reaction: breathing difficulty/
faintness/cool or moist skin/swollen, red, teary
eyes/hives/blotches/swollen nasal passages/
nausea/vomiting/diarrhea (*Very serious reactions
with wheezing and collapse are apt to occur within 5-10 minutes.*)
Less serious: local irritation or pain/moderate
swelling/local redness or itching

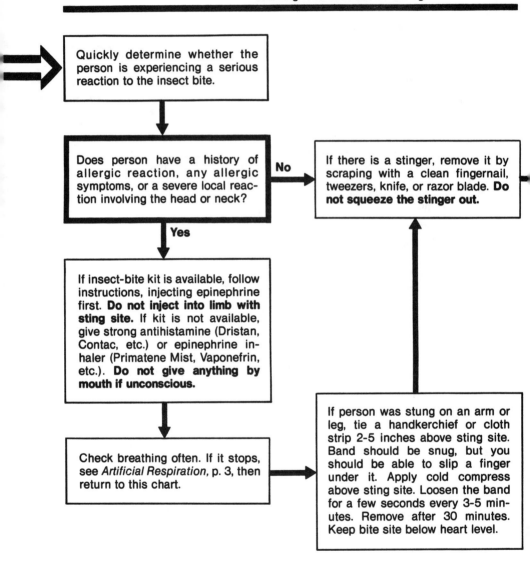

Quickly determine whether the person is experiencing a serious reaction to the insect bite.

Does person have a history of allergic reaction, any allergic symptoms, or a severe local reaction involving the head or neck?

No → If there is a stinger, remove it by scraping with a clean fingernail, tweezers, knife, or razor blade. **Do not squeeze the stinger out.**

Yes

If insect-bite kit is available, follow instructions, injecting epinephrine first. **Do not inject into limb with sting site.** If kit is not available, give strong antihistamine (Dristan, Contac, etc.) or epinephrine inhaler (Primatene Mist, Vaponefrin, etc.). **Do not give anything by mouth if unconscious.**

Check breathing often. If it stops, see *Artificial Respiration,* p. 3, then return to this chart.

If person was stung on an arm or leg, tie a handkerchief or cloth strip 2-5 inches above sting site. Band should be snug, but you should be able to slip a finger under it. Apply cold compress above sting site. Loosen the band for a few seconds every 3-5 minutes. Remove after 30 minutes. Keep bite site below heart level.

Calm the person by talking while attending to the problem. Explain what you are doing. Try not to show concern; act with confidence. Your calm behavior can help to reassure the injured person.

Wash sting site with soap and water. Apply cold compresses for 15-20 minutes, then apply calamine lotion. **Never apply mud.**

For allergic reaction, keep person warm and seek medical care immediately. See *Getting Help,* p. 46. **For minor reaction,** watch for signs of infection or any allergic symptoms that may develop. If they appear, seek medical care. If person is unable to walk, see *Getting Help,* p. 46.

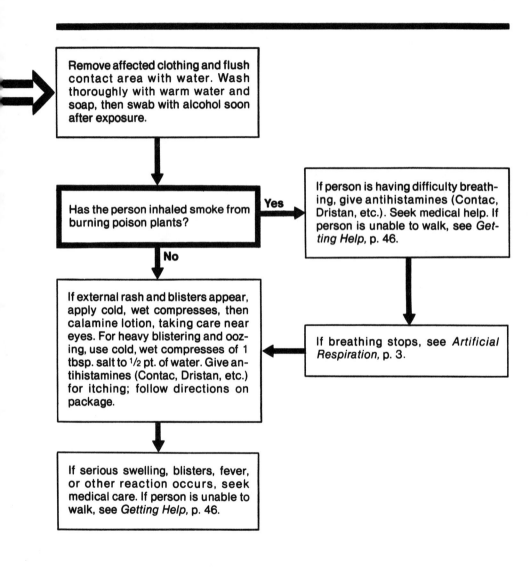

Remove affected clothing and flush contact area with water. Wash thoroughly with warm water and soap, then swab with alcohol soon after exposure.

Has the person inhaled smoke from burning poison plants?

Yes → If person is having difficulty breathing, give antihistamines (Contac, Dristan, etc.). Seek medical help. If person is unable to walk, see *Getting Help*, p. 46.

No

If breathing stops, see *Artificial Respiration*, p. 3.

If external rash and blisters appear, apply cold, wet compresses, then calamine lotion, taking care near eyes. For heavy blistering and oozing, use cold, wet compresses of 1 tbsp. salt to 1/2 pt. of water. Give antihistamines (Contac, Dristan, etc.) for itching; follow directions on package.

If serious swelling, blisters, fever, or other reaction occurs, seek medical care. If person is unable to walk, see *Getting Help*, p. 46.

Calm the person by talking while attending to the problem. Explain what you are doing. Try not to show concern; act with confidence. Your calm behavior can help to reassure the injured person.

Recognize common poison plants:

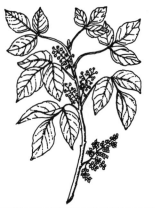

Poison Ivy
Small plant, vine, or shrub common throughout U.S. except California. Shiny leaves grow in clusters of three, turning red and yellow toward Fall.

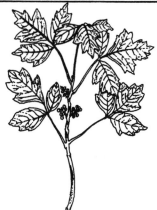

Poison Oak
Western variety grows in California and portions of adjacent states as shrub or vine closely resembling poison ivy.
More common variety grows in other areas, usually as a shrub with clusters of hairy, yellowish berries and undersides of leaves covered with hair.

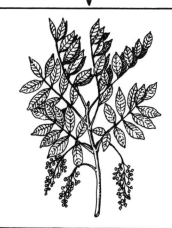

Poison Sumac
Woody shrub or small tree (5-25 feet) grows in eastern U.S., especially in moist climates.
Each leaf stalk has 7-13 leaflets with smooth edges, which turn red in Fall, and cream-colored berries which hang from branches in loose clusters.

These procedures must be followed _immediately_ after snakebite.

Signs & Symptoms:
Poisonous: _Severe reaction occurs within 30 minutes. Burning pain at bite/swelling/discoloration/weakness/dizziness/faint pulse. Coral snake reactions may appear less severe._

Have person lie completely quiet. Keep site of bite below heart level if possible. Remove rings, watch, bracelets.

Apply a light constricting band two inches above bite with a firm wrap from the bite site towards body. Leave it exposed if you have mechanical suction, covered if you do not. Measure the circumference of extremity at site and a couple others to monitor swelling as well as check pulse, color and numbing sensation beyond band. **Do not restrict blood flow.**

Do you have a mechanical suction device such as the Extractor?

Yes

No

Apply suction with a mechanical device such as the Extractor. Incisions will only decrease the amount of venom that can be removed with this device. Applying within the first 5 minutes you can expect up to 35% removal, but further suction can be terminated after 30 minutes, as less than 3% can be expected to be removed.

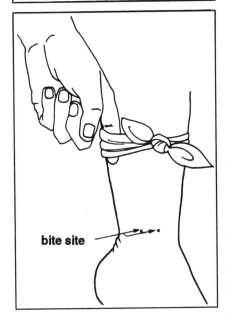

bite site

Calm the person by talking while attending to the problem. Explain what you are doing. Try not to show concern; act with confidence. Your calm behavior can help to reassure the injured person.

Do not "cut and suck", apply cold applications, or give any pain medication. Attempt to identify snake if it doesn't present further danger to others. (See map and description, next page.)

Treat for shock. Seek medical care immediately. (During evacuation, keep the victim from exerting any more energy than is absolutely required.)

Seek medical care at once. See *Getting Help,* p. 46.

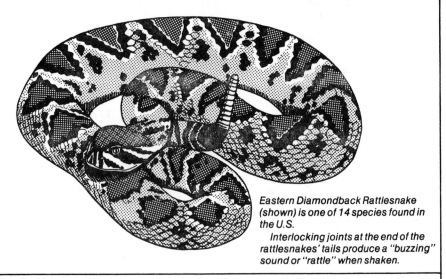

Eastern Diamondback Rattlesnake (shown) is one of 14 species found in the U.S.

Interlocking joints at the end of the rattlesnakes' tails produce a "buzzing" sound or "rattle" when shaken.

Eastern Diamondback Rattlesnake

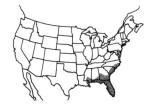

Description Dark diamonds with light borders along a tan or light brown background. Diamonds gradually changing to bands in tail. Diagonal brown lines on the sides of face, vertical on snout.
Habitat Lowland thickets, palmettos, flatwoods.

Canebrake and Timber Rattlesnake

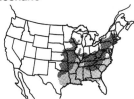

Description South: Dark streak from canebrake snake's eye to mouth; dark chevrons and rusty stripe along midline. Pink to tan ground color darker toward tail, which is black in adults. North: timber rattlesnake has yellowish ground color and a dark phase in part of its range
Habitat Canebrake: lowland brush, and stream borders. Timber rattlesnake: rocky wooded hills.

Western Diamondback Rattlesnake

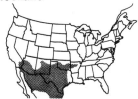

Description Light brown to black diamond-shaped blotches along light grey, tan, and, in some localities, pink background. Black and white bands of about equal width around tail and black basal rattle.
Habitat Diverse terrain: dry, sparsely wooded, rocky hills, flat desert and coastal sand dunes. Often found in agricultural land and near towns.

System

Copperhead

Northern Copperhead (shown here) and other Copperheads in the U.S. vibrate their tails rapidly when alarmed.

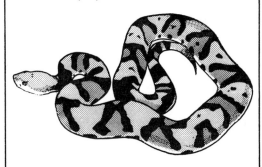

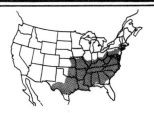

Description Large chestnut brown cross bands on a pale pinkish or reddish-brown surface; and coppery tinge of head.
Habitat North: wooded mountains; hills; wild, damp meadows; along stone walls; in slab or sawdust piles. South: Lowland swamps and uplands; sometimes found in wooded suburbs.

Coral Snakes

Eastern Coral (below) and Texas Coral are dangerously poisonous although their small mouths and short fangs make it difficult to bite most parts of the body.

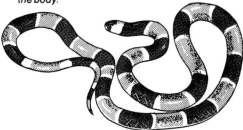

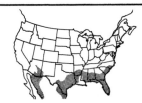

Description Red and black rings, wider than the interspaced yellow rings. Black snout, round pupils; no facial pits.
Habitat East: grassland; dry, open woods; and frequently suburban areas. West: (much less dangerous), desert and semidesert where there is loose soil and rocks.

Cottonmouth (water moccasin)

Eastern Cottonmouth (below), Florida and Western Cottonmouths, are frequently confused with several non-poisonous water snakes.

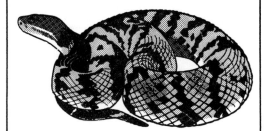

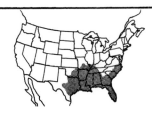

Description Dark blotches on brown or olive body. Heavy body and broad flat head.
Habitat Semiaquatic.

37 Spider or Scorpion Bites
Black Widow, Tarantula, Brown Recluse, Scorpion

Signs & Symptoms: *rigid abdominal muscles without tenderness/breathing difficulty/slurred speech/restlessness/muscle cramps/nausea, vomiting/blister at site/many other possible signs & symptoms.*

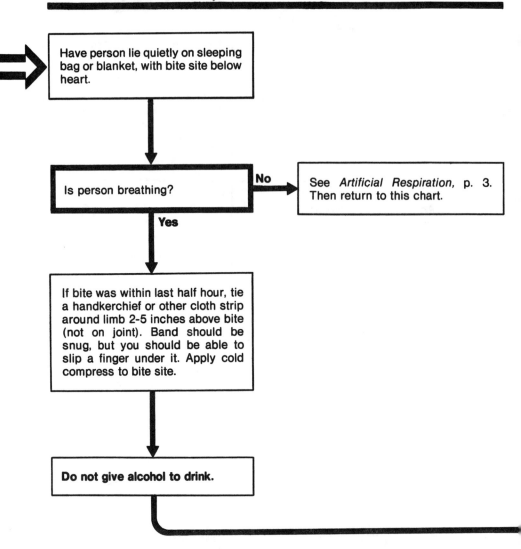

Have person lie quietly on sleeping bag or blanket, with bite site below heart.

Is person breathing? → **No** → See *Artificial Respiration*, p. 3. Then return to this chart.

Yes

If bite was within last half hour, tie a handkerchief or other cloth strip around limb 2-5 inches above bite (not on joint). Band should be snug, but you should be able to slip a finger under it. Apply cold compress to bite site.

Do not give alcohol to drink.

Calm the person by talking while attending to the problem. Explain what you are doing. Try not to show concern; act with confidence. Your calm behavior can help to reassure the injured person.

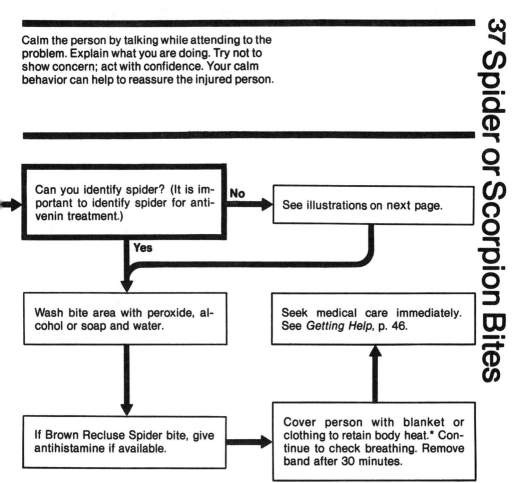

Can you identify spider? (It is important to identify spider for anti-venin treatment.)

No → See illustrations on next page.

Yes ↓

Wash bite area with peroxide, alcohol or soap and water.

Seek medical care immediately. See *Getting Help,* p. 46.

If Brown Recluse Spider bite, give antihistamine if available.

Cover person with blanket or clothing to retain body heat.* Continue to check breathing. Remove band after 30 minutes.

*If weather is very warm and person's skin does not feel cool and clammy, covering will not be necessary.

Black Widow Spider

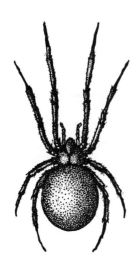

Tarantula

Coal-black, bulbous spider ¾ to 1½ in. long. Bright red hourglass on abdomen. (Be especially cautious in latrines, where these spiders inhabit underside of seats.)

Possible Signs & Symptoms
- sensation of pinprick or minor burning at time of bite
- appearance of small punctures (but sometimes none)
- within 15 to 60 minutes, intense pain at site spreading quickly
- profuse sweating
- rigid abdominal muscles without abdominal tenderness
- other muscle spasms
- breathing difficulty
- slurred speech, poor coordination
- dilated pupils
- generalized swelling of face and extremities

Large, hairy spiders . . . dark brown to black. Up to 7 in. long.

Possible Signs & Symptoms
- may be similar to Black Widow Spider; however, tarantula bites are generally no worse than a bee sting.

Brown Recluse Spider

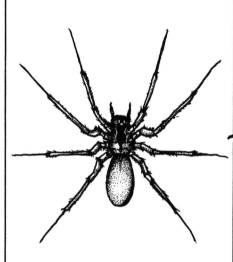

Brownish, rather flat, 1/2-5/8 in. long. Dark brown "violin" on underside. Unlikely in the wilderness; usually found in clothes closets and dark locations in buildings.

Possible Signs & Symptoms
- blister at site
- generalized rash
- joint pain
- chills
- fever
- nausea & vomiting
- pain may become severe after 8 hours

Scorpion

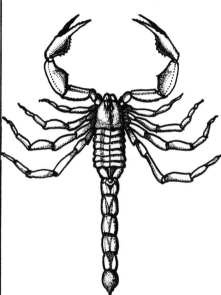

3/4 to 3 in. long. Yellow to greenish-yellow. Lethal variety found only in Arizona and southern California. Night animal. Hides in shoes, boots, sleeping bags.

Possible Signs & Symptoms
- prickling sensation at time of bite, quickly followed by severe pain
- site becomes extremely sensitive
- restlessness
- severe breathing difficulty
- convulsion
- muscle cramps, nausea, vomiting
- high fever
- headache, dizziness
- abdominal pain
- profuse sweating

38 Sprain or Strain

Signs & Symptoms:
Sprain (joint): swelling and discoloration of joint area/pain with movement/no deformity of the joint
Strain (muscle): sharp, tearing pain/possible muscle spasm/possible discoloration (later)/ gradual stiffening of muscle

From the Signs & Symptoms listed above, identify the type of injury.

The injury is a . . .

Sprain

Remove any clothing from around the joint. Elevate the affected joint and support it with rolled blankets, sleeping bag, etc.

Apply cold, wet compresses for 20 minutes every 3-4 hours. Give aspirin or acetaminophen (Tylenol, Datril, etc.). Follow label directions.

Keep the affected joint elevated and continue cold packs for 20 minutes every 3-4 hours.

Do swelling and pain begin to subside after several hours?

No → Continue to keep the injured part immobile. Seek medical care. If person is unable to walk, see *Getting Help*, p. 46.

Yes

After 24 hours, wrap the joint in an elastic bandage, keeping it firm but not too tight. Person should wear this bandage for 3 or 4 days. Apply warm, wet packs to injured area for 20 minutes, 3 times a day.

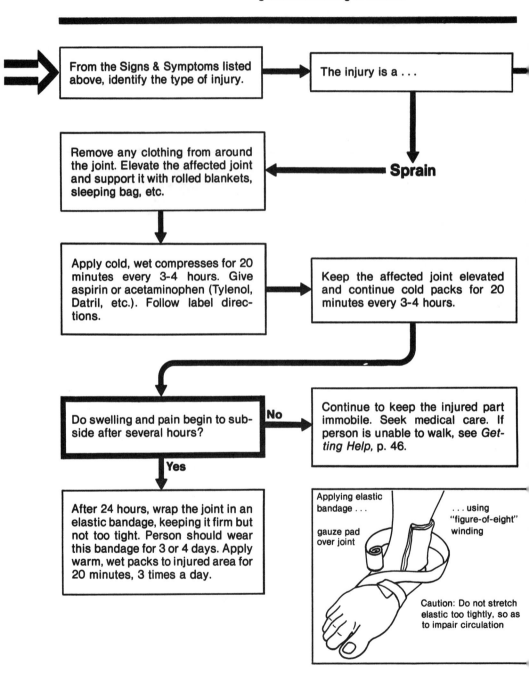

Applying elastic bandage . . .

. . . using "figure-of-eight" winding

gauze pad over joint

Caution: Do not stretch elastic too tightly, so as to impair circulation

Calm the person by talking while attending to the problem. Explain what you are doing. Try not to show concern; act with confidence. Your calm behavior can help to reassure the injured person.

Strain

Is the lower back involved?

Yes → Have the person lie in a comfortable position.

No ↓

Immobilize the affected part by surrounding it with rolled blankets, towels, sleeping bags, etc.

Apply warm, wet packs to the painful area for 20 minutes every 3-4 hours.

Apply cold, wet compresses for 20 minutes every 3-4 hours.

Give aspirin or acetaminophen (Tylenol, Datril, etc.). Follow label directions.

Continue to keep the injured part immobile. If person is unable to walk, see *Getting Help*, p. 46.

No ← Does the pain begin to subside after several hours?

Yes ↓

After 24 hours, apply warm, wet packs for 20 minutes every 3-4 hours. Have the person avoid any activity that produces even minor discomfort for several days.

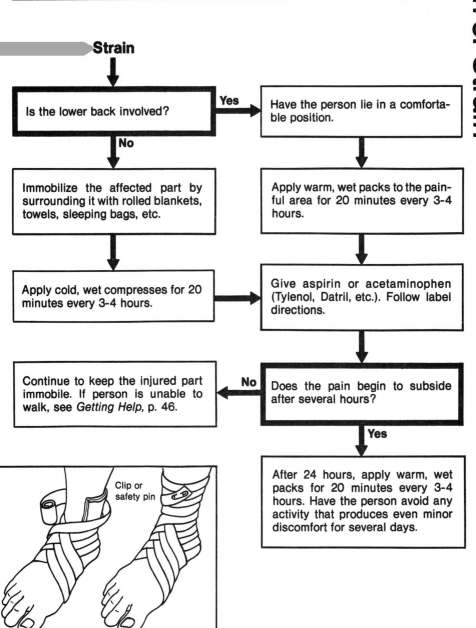

Clip or safety pin

39 Tick Removal

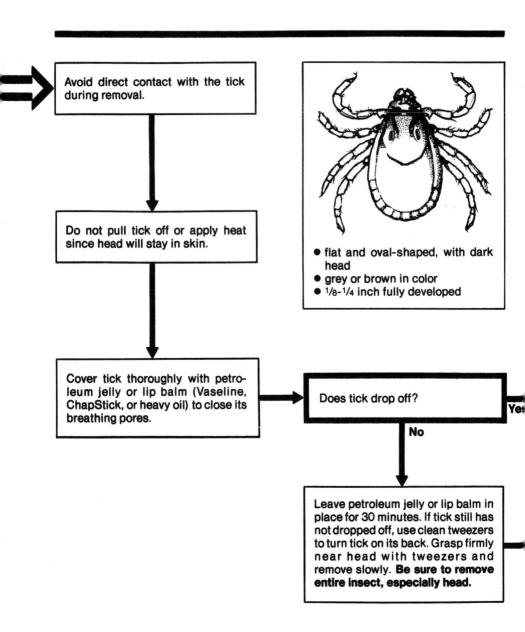

Avoid direct contact with the tick during removal.

Do not pull tick off or apply heat since head will stay in skin.

- flat and oval-shaped, with dark head
- grey or brown in color
- 1/8-1/4 inch fully developed

Cover tick thoroughly with petroleum jelly or lip balm (Vaseline, ChapStick, or heavy oil) to close its breathing pores.

Does tick drop off?

Yes

No

Leave petroleum jelly or lip balm in place for 30 minutes. If tick still has not dropped off, use clean tweezers to turn tick on its back. Grasp firmly near head with tweezers and remove slowly. **Be sure to remove entire insect, especially head.**

Calm the person by talking while attending to the problem. Explain what you are doing. Try not to show concern; act with confidence. Your calm behavior can help to reassure the injured person.

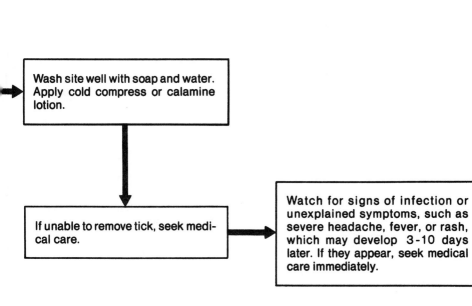

Wash site well with soap and water. Apply cold compress or calamine lotion.

If unable to remove tick, seek medical care.

Watch for signs of infection or unexplained symptoms, such as severe headache, fever, or rash, which may develop 3-10 days later. If they appear, seek medical care immediately.

Definition: *heavy bleeding/involvement of underlying tissues, including muscles, nerves, tendons, or major blood vessels*

Have the person sit or lie in a comfortable position. Immobilize the injured part, if necessary, with rolled blankets or sleeping bag; then elevate it to help reduce bleeding. Cut clothing away from wound.

For other wounds, cover with a thick, sterile gauze pad (or other clean material) and apply gentle, firm, continuous, direct pressure with the palm of your hand.

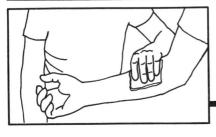

Apply pressure with fingers and thumb to the major artery supplying blood to the wounded area (shown below).

Pressure Points

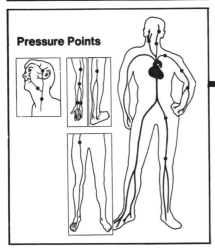

If there is a facial wound, apply finger pressure to the pressure point between wound and heart that is nearest the wound (see pressure points, below left). Use butterfly dressing to close a gaping wound (see *Minor Cuts,* p. 25). Dress with several gauze pads and four-tailed bandage or two bandages crossed and tied at top and back of head. Then see Box A on opposite page.

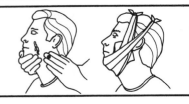

Do not remove the original pad; let blood soak through and begin to clot. If necessary, place additional pads over the original and continue to apply pressure for 5-10 minutes.

Does the bleeding slow down?

No

Does bleeding stop or slow down considerably?

No

Wrap a strip of cloth or other bandage over pad(s). Pull firmly to apply some pressure without cutting off blood circulation. Check position of fingers and thumb and reapply pressure to artery.

Calm the person by talking while attending to the problem. Explain what you are doing. Try not to show concern; act with confidence. Your calm behavior can help to reassure the injured person.

Bleeding Continues

Is the wound on an arm or leg? **No**

Yes

As a last resort, tie a tourniquet just above the wound. Wrap a bandage tightly twice around and turn one end under the other (half-knot). Place any rigid piece of wood on the half-knot and tie one or two additional knots on top. Twist the stick; tighten the tourniquet until bleeding stops. Then tie bar in place with another strip. Once tourniquet is in place, do not loosen or remove.

Bleeding Has Stopped

Leave bandage(s) in place. Add more gauze and strips. Keep affected part elevated. If bandage is very tight, it may be gradually loosened just enough to be more comfortable.

A

If the person has lost a lot of blood, feels faint, or is cold and pale, have him/her lie down. If the wound is not on the head, elevate legs on a rolled blanket or sleeping bag. If there is a head wound, elevate the head slightly. Cover the person with a blanket or clothing to retain body heat.*

If a part has been amputated, save it in cool, fresh water or wrap in clean cloth or towels. If you suspect a fracture, see p. 32.

Watch breathing. If it stops, see *Artificial Respiration,* p. 3.

Seek medical care immediately. See *Getting Help,* p. 46.

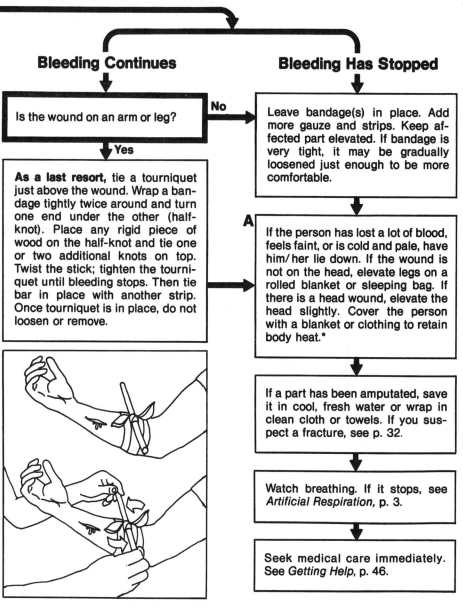

*If weather is very warm and person's skin does not feel cool and clammy, covering will not be necessary.

41 Cold Exposure

Signs & Symptoms: *low body temperature/ uncontrollable shivering/poor muscle coordination/shallow breathing/mental confusion/ drowsiness/numbness/possible loss of consciousness*

If there is more than one rescuer, one should go for help while the other is aiding the injured person.

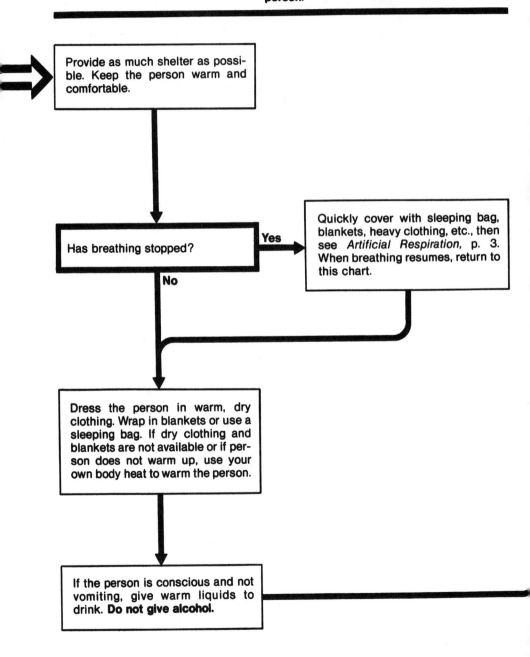

Provide as much shelter as possible. Keep the person warm and comfortable.

Has breathing stopped?

Yes → Quickly cover with sleeping bag, blankets, heavy clothing, etc., then see *Artificial Respiration,* p. 3. When breathing resumes, return to this chart.

No

Dress the person in warm, dry clothing. Wrap in blankets or use a sleeping bag. If dry clothing and blankets are not available or if person does not warm up, use your own body heat to warm the person.

If the person is conscious and not vomiting, give warm liquids to drink. **Do not give alcohol.**

Calm the person by talking while attending to the problem. Explain what you are doing. Try not to show concern; act with confidence. Your calm behavior can help to reassure the injured person.

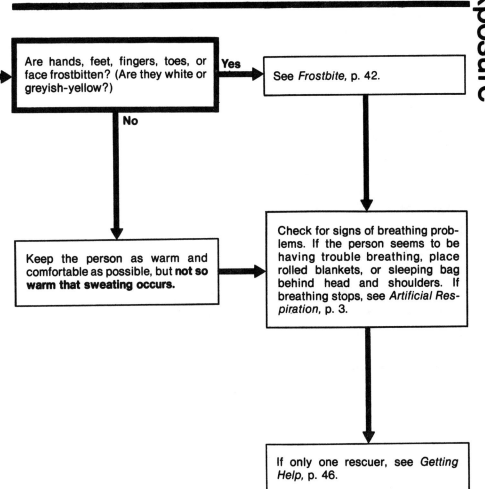

Are hands, feet, fingers, toes, or face frostbitten? (Are they white or greyish-yellow?)

Yes → See *Frostbite*, p. 42.

No

Keep the person as warm and comfortable as possible, but **not so warm that sweating occurs.**

Check for signs of breathing problems. If the person seems to be having trouble breathing, place rolled blankets, or sleeping bag behind head and shoulders. If breathing stops, see *Artificial Respiration*, p. 3.

If only one rescuer, see *Getting Help*, p. 46.

42Frostbite

Signs & Symptoms: *possible pain in early stage/skin white or grayish-yellow/extreme coldness and numbness of affected part/possible blisters*

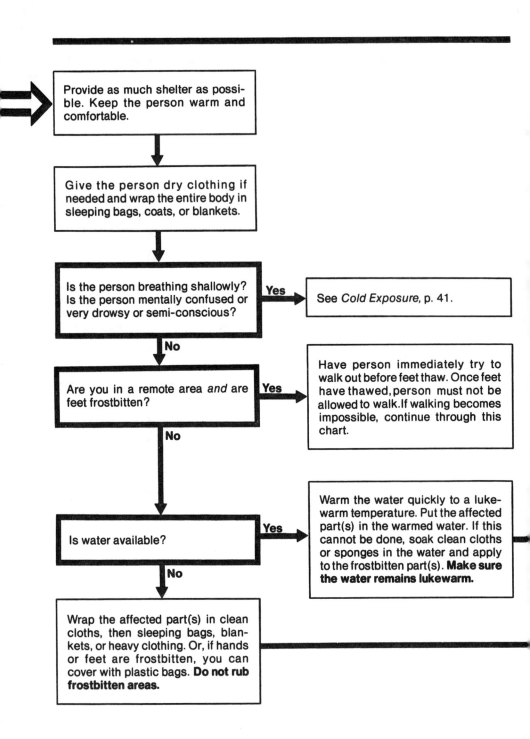

Provide as much shelter as possible. Keep the person warm and comfortable.

Give the person dry clothing if needed and wrap the entire body in sleeping bags, coats, or blankets.

Is the person breathing shallowly? Is the person mentally confused or very drowsy or semi-conscious? — **Yes** → See *Cold Exposure,* p. 41.

No

Are you in a remote area *and* are feet frostbitten? — **Yes** → Have person immediately try to walk out before feet thaw. Once feet have thawed, person must not be allowed to walk. If walking becomes impossible, continue through this chart.

No

Is water available? — **Yes** → Warm the water quickly to a lukewarm temperature. Put the affected part(s) in the warmed water. If this cannot be done, soak clean cloths or sponges in the water and apply to the frostbitten part(s). **Make sure the water remains lukewarm.**

No

Wrap the affected part(s) in clean cloths, then sleeping bags, blankets, or heavy clothing. Or, if hands or feet are frostbitten, you can cover with plastic bags. **Do not rub frostbitten areas.**

Calm the person by talking while attending to the problem. Explain what you are doing. Try not to show concern; act with confidence. Your calm behavior can help to reassure the injured person.

Continue rewarming until the affected part becomes flushed. Then discontinue. Have the person move the part. If *feet* were frostbitten, do *not* allow the person to walk.

If fingers or toes were frostbitten, dry carefully without rubbing. Separate those affected with dry, sterile gauze or clean cloth. Elevate affected part(s) and protect from direct contact with bedclothes or other materials.

Keep the person sheltered from the cold and as warm and comfortable as possible, but **not so warm that sweating occurs.**

Give the person warm liquids to drink. **Do not give alcoholic beverages. Do not let person smoke.**

Keep the person away from sources of direct heat. If there are blisters, do not break them.

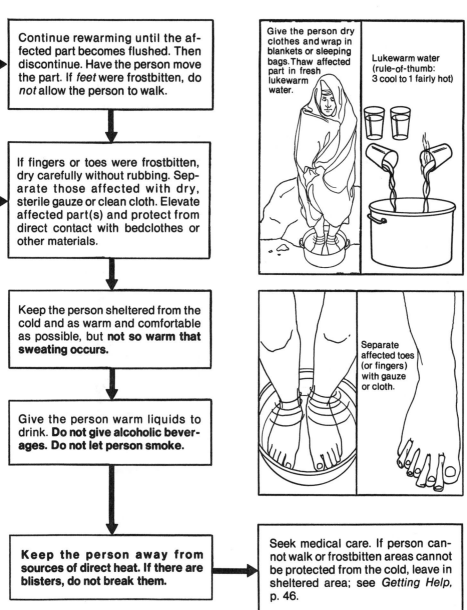

Give the person dry clothes and wrap in blankets or sleeping bags. Thaw affected part in fresh lukewarm water.

Lukewarm water (rule-of-thumb: 3 cool to 1 fairly hot)

Separate affected toes (or fingers) with gauze or cloth.

Seek medical care. If person cannot walk or frostbitten areas cannot be protected from the cold, leave in sheltered area; see *Getting Help*, p. 46.

43 Heat Exhaustion/ Heat Cramps

Signs & Symptoms: *cold, pale, clammy skin/fatigue and faintness/headache/ heavy sweating/weak pulse/near-normal body temperature/nausea/ gradual onset*

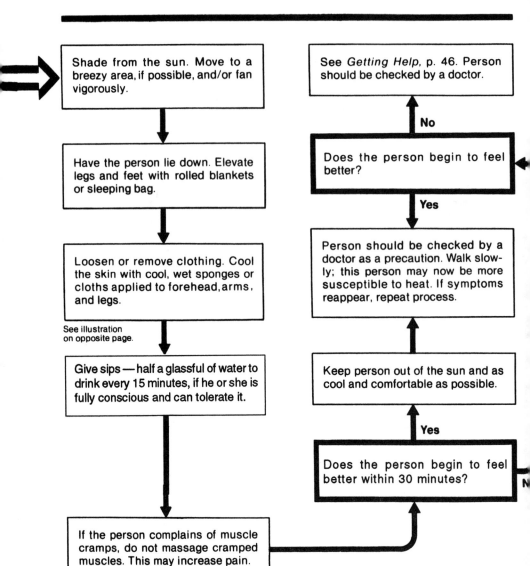

Shade from the sun. Move to a breezy area, if possible, and/or fan vigorously.

Have the person lie down. Elevate legs and feet with rolled blankets or sleeping bag.

Loosen or remove clothing. Cool the skin with cool, wet sponges or cloths applied to forehead, arms, and legs.

See illustration on opposite page.

Give sips — half a glassful of water to drink every 15 minutes, if he or she is fully conscious and can tolerate it.

If the person complains of muscle cramps, do not massage cramped muscles. This may increase pain.

See *Getting Help*, p. 46. Person should be checked by a doctor.

No

Does the person begin to feel better?

Yes

Person should be checked by a doctor as a precaution. Walk slowly; this person may now be more susceptible to heat. If symptoms reappear, repeat process.

Keep person out of the sun and as cool and comfortable as possible.

Yes

Does the person begin to feel better within 30 minutes?

N

Calm the person by talking while attending to the problem. Explain what you are doing. Try not to show concern; act with confidence. Your calm behavior can help to reassure the sick person.

If any of these occur, see *Heat-stroke,* p. 44.

Yes

No Does temperature suddenly rise? Are there convulsions, stupor, or unconsciousness?

Continue cooling with wet cloths. Check body temperature every 5 minutes for 1/2 hour.

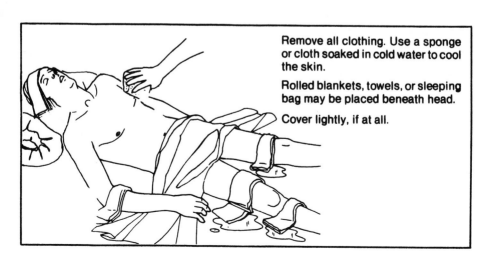

Remove all clothing. Use a sponge or cloth soaked in cold water to cool the skin.

Rolled blankets, towels, or sleeping bag may be placed beneath head.

Cover lightly, if at all.

44 Heatstroke

Signs & Symptoms: *red, hot, dry skin/no perspiration/body temperature around 106°F (or very warm to the touch)/strong rapid pulse/stupor or unconsciousness*

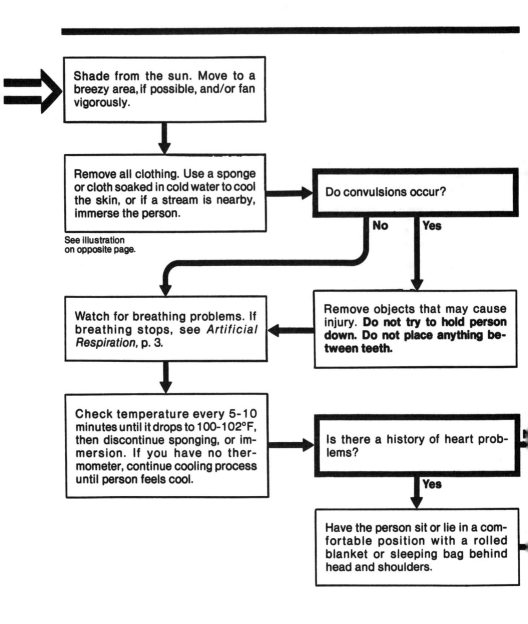

Shade from the sun. Move to a breezy area, if possible, and/or fan vigorously.

Remove all clothing. Use a sponge or cloth soaked in cold water to cool the skin, or if a stream is nearby, immerse the person.

See illustration
on opposite page.

Do convulsions occur?

No   Yes

Watch for breathing problems. If breathing stops, see *Artificial Respiration*, p. 3.

Remove objects that may cause injury. **Do not try to hold person down. Do not place anything between teeth.**

Check temperature every 5-10 minutes until it drops to 100-102°F, then discontinue sponging, or immersion. If you have no thermometer, continue cooling process until person feels cool.

Is there a history of heart problems?

Yes

Have the person sit or lie in a comfortable position with a rolled blanket or sleeping bag behind head and shoulders.

Calm the person by talking while attending to the problem. Explain what you are doing. Try not to show concern; act with confidence. Your calm behavior can help to reassure the sick person.

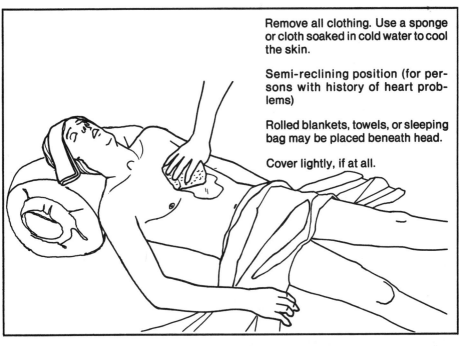

Remove all clothing. Use a sponge or cloth soaked in cold water to cool the skin.

Semi-reclining position (for persons with history of heart problems)

Rolled blankets, towels, or sleeping bag may be placed beneath head.

Cover lightly, if at all.

Have the person lie flat. *Do not* cover unless chilled. Then cover lightly.

This person must receive medical care. If there is only one rescuer, see *Getting Help,* p. 46.

Continue to shade from the sun and keep as cool and comfortable as possible. Continue to watch breathing. Check temperature every 15 minutes for one hour.

If temperature begins to rise again, repeat the cooling process.

45 High Altitude Illness

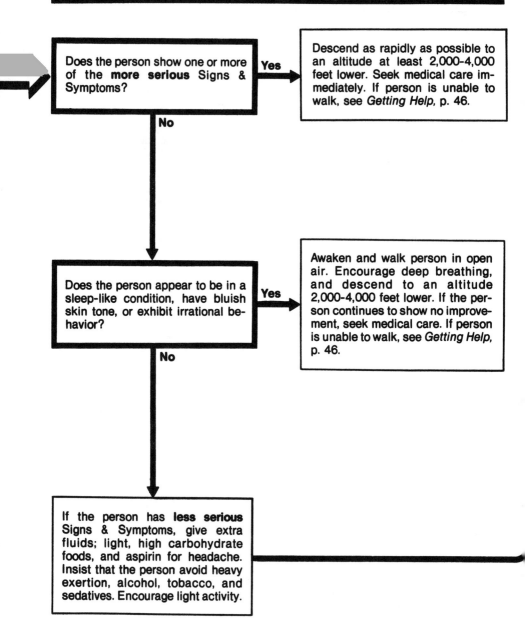

Does the person show one or more of the **more serious** Signs & Symptoms?

Yes → Descend as rapidly as possible to an altitude at least 2,000-4,000 feet lower. Seek medical care immediately. If person is unable to walk, see *Getting Help,* p. 46.

No ↓

Does the person appear to be in a sleep-like condition, have bluish skin tone, or exhibit irrational behavior?

Yes → Awaken and walk person in open air. Encourage deep breathing, and descend to an altitude 2,000-4,000 feet lower. If the person continues to show no improvement, seek medical care. If person is unable to walk, see *Getting Help,* p. 46.

No ↓

If the person has **less serious** Signs & Symptoms, give extra fluids; light, high carbohydrate foods, and aspirin for headache. Insist that the person avoid heavy exertion, alcohol, tobacco, and sedatives. Encourage light activity.

Calm the person by talking while attending to the problem. Explain what you are doing. Try not to show concern; act with confidence. Your calm behavior can help to reassure the sick person.

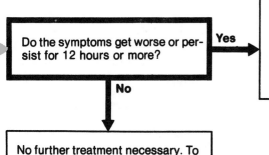

Do the symptoms get worse or persist for 12 hours or more?

Yes → Descend to an altitude at least 2,000-4,000 feet lower. If person continues to show no improvement, seek medical care. If person is unable to walk, see *Getting Help*, p. 46.

No → No further treatment necessary. To prevent future attacks, ascend gradually, and avoid heavy exertion for 2-3 days after reaching high altitude.

46 Getting Help

The following charts will aid you in deciding whether a person can walk to help, whether he or she can be left alone, and what precautions you should take before heading for assistance. Give all medical care indicated in the emergency procedure charts, and be sure the person's condition is stable before going for help.

Index

If a person is unable to walk and must be left alone, use *Distress Signals,* (see p. i) and mark your trail (see p. ii).

Back & Neck Injuries 1 rescuer	G3
Back & Neck Injuries 2 or more rescuers	G4
Bruise shock symptoms, coughing up blood, or bleeding from rectum	G5
Bruise extensive, increasing in size	G6
Burns second and third degree	H1
Chemical Poisoning convulsions	H2
Chemical Poisoning unconsciousness	H3
Chemical Poisoning	H4
Chest Injury sucking wound	H5
Chest Injury section of chest wall moving differently than normal	H6
Chest Injury section of chest sunken, or frothy blood coming from mouth	I1
Chest Injury no outward signs of injury, but chest pain and abdominal pain	I2
Minor Cuts gaping wound	I3
Minor Cuts signs of infection	I4
Dislocations jaw	I5
Dislocations shoulder, elbow, wrist, finger	I6
Dislocations hip, knee, ankle, etc.	I7
Chemical Burns of the Eyes	J1
Foreign Object in Eye discoloration, swelling, or pain	J2
Foreign Object in Eye cornea	J3

Eye Injury foreign object	J4
Eye Injury bleeding wound	J5
Eye Injury pain, blurred vision, swelling, other symptoms	J6
Fishhook Removal imbedded fishhook near eyes, ears, nose, or groin	J7
Fishhook Removal imbedded fishhook without shearing device	K1
Food Poisoning	K2
Fractures limb	K3
Severe Head Injury	K4
Insect Sting allergic reaction	K5
Poison Ivy, Oak, or Sumac serious swelling, blisters, fever, other reactions	K6
Snakebite	L1
Spider Bites	L2
Sprain or Strain sprain with swelling for more than several hours	L3
Sprain or Strain strain with pain for more than several hours	L4
Deep Wound	L5

Exposure to Heat, Cold, or Altitude

Problem	See
Cold Exposure	L6
Frostbite	M1
Heat Exhaustion/Heat Cramps	M2
Heatstroke	M3
High Altitude Illness	M4

A Getting Help

A Problem	If necessary, can person walk for help? Any precautions?	Can person be left alone?	If left alone, what precautions should be taken?
1 **Artificial Respiration** Person doesn't revive in 30 minutes.	No	No See *Distress Signals*, p.i.	
2 **Artificial Respiration** Person revives, but breathing difficulty unknown.	Yes, if able to walk. Precautions: Walk slowly.	No, unless no other way to get help and person appears to be breathing adequately.	See *Distress Signals*, p.i. Set up shelter. Protect person from direct contact with ground if possible. Cover with shirt, jacket, sweater, etc., to keep in body heat. Leave food and water.
3 **Choking**	No	No See *Distress Signals*, p.i.	
4 **CPR** (1 rescuer)	No	No See *Distress Signals*, p.i.	
5 **CPR** (2 or more rescuers)	No	No See *Distress Signals*, p.i.	
6 **CPR** (Infants)	No	No See *Distress Signals*, p.i.	
7 **Abdominal Pain** Sharp or burning pain in mid-upper abdominal region with pain radiating to arm(s), neck, or jaw; difficulty breathing; pale or bluish skin, lips or nails	No	No, unless no other way to get help.	See *Distress Signals*, p.i. Set up shelter. Protect person from direct contact with ground if possible. Cover with shirt, jacket, sweater, etc., to keep in body heat. Make sure person is comfortable.

B	Problem	If necessary, can person walk for help? Any precautions?	Can person be left alone?	If left alone, what precautions should be taken?
1	**Abdominal Pain** Sharp or burning pain in mid-upper abdominal region	No	Yes	Set up shelter. Protect person from direct contact with ground if possible. Cover with shirt, jacket, sweater, etc., to keep in body heat. Make sure person is comfortable.
2	**Abdominal Pain** with rigid abdomen, vomiting blood, or bloody diarrhea	No	No, unless no other way to get help.	See *Distress Signals*, p.i. Set up shelter. Protect person from direct contact with ground if possible. Cover with shirt, jacket, sweater, etc., to keep in body heat. Make sure person is comfortable.
3	**Abdominal Pain** persisting	Yes, if able to walk. Precautions: Walk slowly. Rest often.	Yes, but only if necessary.	Set up shelter. Protect person from direct contact with ground if possible. Cover with shirt, jacket, sweater, etc., to keep in body heat. Make sure person is comfortable.
4	**Chest Pain** Intense, squeezing, constricting pain possibly radiating to neck, jaw, shoulder(s), arm(s); nausea; vomiting; cold sweats; breathing difficulty	No	No See *Distress Signals*, p.i.	
5	**Chest Pain** lasting more than 1 hour	No	Yes, but only if necessary.	See *Distress Signals*, p.i. Set up shelter. Protect person from direct contact with ground if possible. Leave plenty of fluids. **No alcohol. No salty liquids such as broth** if breathing difficulties.
6	**Chest Pain** lasting more than 1 hour with respiratory infection	Yes, if able to walk.	Yes, but only if necessary.	Set up shelter. Protect person from direct contact with ground, if possible. Leave plenty of fluids. **No alcohol. No salty liquids such as broth** if breathing difficulties.

C	Problem	If necessary, can person walk for help? Any precautions?	Can person be left alone?	If left alone, what precautions should be taken?
1	**Convulsion**	Yes, after 2-3 hours of rest and person appears to be back to normal.	Yes, but only if necessary, and only after person appears to have recovered from the convulsion.	Set up shelter. Protect person from direct contact with ground if possible. Cover with shirt, jacket, sweater, etc., to keep in body heat. Loosen tight fitting clothing. Leave food and water.
2	**Diabetic Emergencies** Diabetic coma	No	No, unless no other way to get help.	See *Distress Signals*, p.i. Set up shelter. Protect person from direct contact with ground if possible. Make sure person is comfortable.
3	**Diabetic Emergencies** Insulin shock with unconsciousness	No	No, unless no other way to get help or condition is under control.	See *Distress Signals*, p.i. Set up shelter. Protect person from direct contact with ground if possible. Cover with shirt, jacket, sweater, etc., to keep in body heat. Make sure person is comfortable.
4	**Diabetic Emergencies** Insulin shock with convulsion	No	No, unless no other way to get help or condition is under control.	See *Distress Signals*, p.i. Set up shelter. Protect person from direct contact with ground if possible. Cover with shirt, jacket, sweater, etc., to keep in body heat. Make sure person is comfortable.
5	**Fever** with urinary tract infection	Yes, if able to walk. If too weak to walk, make an Indian sled (travois). Precautions: Walk slowly. Make a walking stick for support.	Yes, if fever is under control.	Set up shelter. Protect person from direct contact with ground if possible. Give plenty of fluids. **(No alcohol.)** Try to lower temperature with cool, wet cloths before leaving.

D Problem

#	Problem	If necessary, can person walk for help? Any precautions?	Can person be left alone?	If left alone, what precautions should be taken?
1	**Fever** with headache and stiff neck	Yes, but only if necessary. Precautions: Walk slowly. Make a walking stick for support. Rest often.	Yes, but only if necessary.	Set up shelter. Protect person from direct contact with ground if possible. Give plenty of fluids. **(No alcohol.)** Try to lower temperature with cool, wet cloths before leaving.
2	**Fever** with shock symptoms	No	No, unless condition is under control.	See *Distress Signals*, p.i. Set up shelter. Protect person from direct contact with ground if possible. Cover with shirt, jacket, sweater, etc., to keep in body heat. Make sure person is comfortable. Leave fluids.
3	**Fever** of 102° or higher for more than 6 hours	Yes, but only if necessary.	No, unless no other way to reach help or temperature comes down.	See *Distress Signals*, p.i. Set up shelter. Protect person from direct contact with ground if possible. Give plenty of fluids. **(No alcohol.)** Try to lower temperature with cool, wet cloths before leaving. Elevate legs with rolled sleeping bag. Cover with shirt, jacket, sweater, etc., to keep in body heat.
4	**Headache** with numbness or weakness in hands or feet, slurred speech, or breathing difficulty	No	No, unless no other way to get help.	See *Distress Signals*, p.i. Set up shelter. Protect person from direct contact with ground if possible. Cover with shirt, jacket, sweater, etc., to keep in body heat. Make person comfortable.
5	**Headache** that continues for more than 4 hours or gets worse	Yes, if able to walk.	No, unless no other way to get help.	See *Distress Signals*, p.i. Set up shelter. Protect person from direct contact with ground if possible. Cover with shirt, jacket, sweater, etc., to keep in body heat. Leave food and water. Make sure person is comfortable.

E	Problem	If necessary, can person walk for help? Any precautions?	Can person be left alone?	If left alone, what precautions should be taken?
1	**Nausea & Vomiting** Pregnant woman with nausea & vomiting	Yes, if able to walk. Precaution: Walk slowly.	Yes	Set up shelter. Protect person from direct contact with ground if possible. Make sure person is comfortable.
2	**Nausea & Vomiting** Vomit is black or bloody.	Yes, if able to walk. Precaution: Do not give anything to eat or drink.	Yes	Set up shelter. Protect person from direct contact with ground if possible. Make sure person is comfortable.
3	**Nausea & Vomiting** Black or bloody diarrhea	Yes, if able to walk. Precaution: Do not give anything to eat or drink.	Yes	Set up shelter. Protect person from direct contact with ground if possible. Make sure person is comfortable.
4	**Nausea & Vomiting** for more than 1 hour	Yes, if able to walk. Precautions: Walk slowly. Rest often.	Yes	Set up shelter. Protect person from direct contact with ground if possible. Make sure person is comfortable.
5	**Nosebleed** with uncontrolled bleeding	Yes, after bleeding slows down or stops.	Yes	Set up shelter. Protect person from direct contact with ground if possible. Cover with shirt, jacket, sweater, etc., to keep in body heat. Make sure person is comfortable.
6	**Nosebleed** with a suspected fracture	Yes, if able to walk. Precautions: Walk slowly. Stop if bleeding becomes uncontrollable.	Yes	Set up shelter. Protect person from direct contact with ground if possible. Cover with shirt, jacket, sweater etc., to keep in body heat. Make sure person is comfortable.

F Problem

	Problem	If necessary, can person walk for help? Any precautions?	Can person be left alone?	If left alone, what precautions should be taken?
1	**Unconsciousness** with a history of heart problems	No	No See *Distress Signals*, p.l.	
2	**Unconsciousness** lasting more than a few minutes	No	No, unless no other way to get help.	See *Distress Signals*, p.l. Set up shelter. Protect person from direct contact with ground if possible. Cover with shirt, jacket, sweater, etc., to keep in body heat. Make sure person is comfortable.
3	**Abdominal Injury** with suspected hernia	Yes, if able to walk. Precautions: Bandage hernia tightly with bandana or similar material to hold with tips of fingers. Walk slowly. Make a walking stick for support.	Yes	Set up shelter. Protect person from direct contact with ground if possible. Cover with shirt, jacket, sweater, etc., to keep in body heat. Make sure person is comfortable.
4	**Abdominal Injury** with internal bleeding	No	No, unless no other way to get help.	See *Distress Signals*, p.l. Set up shelter. Protect person from direct contact with ground if possible. Make sure person is comfortable.
5	**Abdominal Injury** with protruding organs	No	No See *Distress Signals*, p.l.	
6	**Abdominal Injury** with foreign object penetrating abdomen	No	No See *Distress Signals*, p.l.	

G Problem

	Problem	If necessary, can person walk for help? Any precautions?	Can person be left alone?	If left alone, what precautions should be taken?
1	**Abdominal Injury**	Yes, if able to walk. Precaution: Walk slowly and cautiously.	No. unless no other way to get help.	See *Distress Signals*, p.i. Set up shelter. Protect person from direct contact with ground if possible. Make sure person is comfortable.
2	**Animal Bites**	Yes, if able to walk.	Yes, after bleeding has stopped.	Set up shelter. Protect person from direct contact with ground if possible. Make sure person is comfortable. Leave food and water.
3	**Back & Neck Injuries** with 1 rescuer	No	Yes, but only if necessary.	Set up shelter. Protect person from direct contact with ground if possible. Immobilize back and neck. Cover with shirt, jacket, sweater, etc., to keep in body heat. Leave food and water.
4	**Back & Neck Injuries** with 2 or more rescuers	No	Yes, but only if necessary.	If a rescuer is left with person, follow instructions in box above.
5	**Bruise** with shock symptoms, coughing up blood, or bleeding from rectum	No	Yes, after bleeding stops and condition is under control.	Set up shelter. Protect person from direct contact with ground if possible. Cover with shirt, jacket, sweater, etc., to keep in body heat. Make sure person is comfortable.
6	**Bruise** Extensive; increasing in size	Yes, if able to walk. Precautions: Walk slowly. Make a crutch or walking stick if a leg bruise.	Yes	Set up shelter. Protect person from direct contact with ground if possible. Cover with shirt, jacket, sweater, etc., to keep in body heat. Leave cold compresses to apply to bruise.

H Problem

#	Problem	If necessary, can person walk for help? Any precautions?	Can person be left alone?	If left alone, what precautions should be taken?
1	**Burns** Second & Third degree	Yes, if able to walk.	No, unless no other way to get help.	See *Distress Signals*, p.i. Set up shelter. Protect person from direct contact with ground if possible. Cover with shirt, jacket, sweater, etc., to keep in body heat. Make sure person is comfortable.
2	**Chemical Poisoning** with convulsions	No	No, unless condition is under control and convulsions stop.	See *Distress Signals*, p.i. Set up shelter. Protect person from direct contact with ground if possible. Cover with shirt, jacket, sweater, etc., to keep in body heat. Make sure person is comfortable.
3	**Chemical Poisoning** with unconsciousness	No	No, unless no other way to get help.	See *Distress Signals*, p.i. Set up shelter. Protect person from direct contact with ground if possible. Cover with shirt, jacket, sweater, etc., to keep in body heat. Make sure person is comfortable. Turn head to side.
4	**Chemical Poisoning**	Yes, if able to walk.	Yes, if condition is under control.	Set up shelter. Protect person from direct contact with ground if possible. Cover with shirt, jacket, sweater, etc., to keep in body heat. Make sure person is comfortable.
5	**Chest Injury** with a sucking wound	Yes, if able to walk.	Yes, but only if necessary.	See *Distress Signals*, p.i. Set up shelter. Protect person from direct contact with ground if possible. Make sure person is comfortable.
6	**Chest Injury** with a section of chest wall moving differently than normal	No	No See *Distress Signals*, p.i.	

Getting Help

	Problem	If necessary, can person walk for help? Any precautions?	Can person be left alone?	If left alone, what precautions should be taken?
1	**Chest Injury** with a section of chest sunken or frothy blood coming from mouth	No	No *See Distress Signals*, p.l.	
2	**Chest Injury** with no outward signs of injury, but person has chest and abdominal pain	No	No *See Distress Signals*, p.l.	
3	**Minor Cuts** with gaping wound	Yes, if able to walk.	Yes	Set up shelter. Protect person from direct contact with ground if possible. Make sure person is comfortable. Leave food and water.
4	**Minor Cuts** with signs of infection	Yes, if able to walk.	Yes	Set up shelter. Protect person from direct contact with ground if possible. Make sure person is comfortable. Leave food and water.
5	**Dislocations** Jaw	Yes Precaution: Immobilize jaw.	Yes	Set up shelter. Protect person from direct contact with ground if possible. Leave fluids and soft foods.
6	**Dislocations** Shoulder, elbow, wrist, finger	Yes, if able to walk.	Yes	Set up shelter. Protect person from direct contact with ground if possible. Make sure person is comfortable. Leave food and water.
7	**Dislocations** Hip, knee, ankle, etc.	Yes, only if necessary and able to walk. Precautions: Walk slowly. Use strong stick for support to keep weight off injured area.	Yes, but only if necessary.	Set up shelter. Protect person from direct contact with ground if possible. Leave fluids and food. Immobilize injury.

J Problem

	Problem	If necessary, can person walk for help? Any precautions?	Can person be left alone?	If left alone, what precautions should be taken?
1	**Chemical Burns of the Eyes**	Yes, if able to walk.	Yes, if some vision remains.	Set up shelter. Protect person from direct contact with ground if possible. Make sure person is comfortable. Leave food and water.
2	**Foreign Object in Eye** with discoloration, swelling, or pain	Yes, if able to walk.	Yes	Set up shelter. Protect person from direct contact with ground if possible. Make sure person is comfortable. Leave food and water.
3	**Foreign Object** in cornea	Yes, if able to walk.	Yes	Set up shelter. Protect person from direct contact with ground if possible. Make sure person is comfortable. Leave food and water.
4	**Eye Injury** with foreign object	No	Yes	Set up shelter. Protect person from direct contact with ground if possible. Make sure person is comfortable. Leave food and water.
5	**Eye Injury** with bleeding wound	Yes, if able to walk, and after bleeding is controlled.	Yes	Set up shelter. Protect person from direct contact with ground if possible. Make sure person is comfortable. Leave food and water.
6	**Eye Injury** with pain, blurred vision, swelling, or other similar symptoms	Yes, if someone can guide person and person is able to walk.	Yes, but only if necessary.	Set up shelter. Protect person from direct contact with ground if possible. Cover with shirt, jacket, sweater, etc., to keep in body heat. Leave food and water.
7	**Fishhook Removal** Imbedded fishhook near eyes, ears, nose, or groin	Yes, if able to walk. Precaution: Walk slowly.	Yes	Set up shelter. Protect person from direct contact with ground if possible. Cover with shirt, jacket, sweater, etc., to keep in body heat. Make sure hook doesn't move and person is comfortable. Leave food and water.

K	Problem	If necessary, can person walk for help? Any precautions?	Can person be left alone?	If left alone, what precautions should be taken?
1	**Fishhook Removal** Imbedded fishhook without shearing device to remove it.	Yes, if able to walk.	Yes	Set up shelter. Protect person from direct contact with ground if possible. Cover with shirt, jacket, sweater, etc., to keep in body heat. Make sure hook doesn't move and person is comfortable. Leave food and water.
2	**Food Poisoning**	Yes, if strong enough to walk.	Yes, but only if necessary.	Set up shelter. Protect person from direct contact with ground if possible. Give plenty of fluids. Cover with shirt, jacket, sweater, etc., to keep in body heat. Make sure person is comfortable.
3	**Fracture** limb	Yes, if able to walk.	Yes	Set up shelter. Protect person from direct contact with ground if possible. Cover with shirt, jacket, sweater, etc., to keep in body heat. Leave food and water. Make person comfortable.
4	**Severe Head Injury**	Yes, if able to walk.	No, unless no other way to get help.	See *Distress Signals*, p.i. Set up shelter. Protect person from direct contact with ground if possible. Cover with shirt, jacket, sweater, etc., to keep in body heat. Make person comfortable.
5	**Insect Sting** with allergic reaction	Yes, after condition is under control, and if able to walk.	Yes	Set up shelter. Protect person from direct contact with ground if possible. Cover with shirt, jacket, sweater, etc., to keep in body heat. Make sure person is comfortable. Leave water.
6	**Poison Ivy, Oak, or Sumac** with serious swelling, blisters,	Yes, if able to walk.	Yes	Set up shelter. Protect person from direct contact with ground if possible. Make sure person is comfortable. Leave food and water.

L Problem

	Problem	If necessary, can person walk for help? Any precautions?	Can person be left alone?	If left alone, what precautions should be taken?
1	**Snakebite**	Yes, unless poisonous snakebite.	Yes	Set up shelter. Protect person from direct contact with ground if possible. Make sure person is comfortable. Leave food and water.
2	**Spider Bites**	Yes, if able to walk.	Yes	Set up shelter. Protect person from direct contact with ground if possible. Make sure person is comfortable. Leave food and water.
3	**Sprain or Strain** Sprain with swelling and pain for more than several hours	Yes, if able to walk. Precaution: Make a walking stick for support.	Yes	Set up shelter. Protect person from direct contact with ground if possible. Make sure person is comfortable. Leave food and water.
4	**Sprain or Strain** Strain with pain for more than several hours	Yes, if able to walk. Precaution: Make a walking stick for support.	Yes	Set up shelter. Protect person from direct contact with ground if possible. Make sure person is comfortable. Leave food and water.
5	**Deep Wound**	Yes, if able to walk, and after bleeding is controlled.	Yes, after bleeding has stopped.	Set up shelter. Protect person from direct contact with ground if possible. Bleeding should be controlled. Leave food and water.
6	**Cold Exposure**	No, unless person is warmed up and condition is under control.	No, unless person is warmed up and condition is under control.	See *Distress Signals*, p.I. Set up shelter. Protect person from direct contact with ground if possible. Leave fluids and food. Make sure person is warm.

M Problem

	Problem	If necessary, can person walk for help? Any precautions?	Can person be left alone?	If left alone, what precautions should be taken?
1	Frostbite	Yes, if feet were not affected. Precautions: Protect injured parts from cold. If feet were affected, person must not walk once feet have begun to thaw.	Yes	Set up shelter to protect from the wind. Protect person from direct contact with ground if possible. Leave fluids and food. Make sure person is comfortable.
2	Heat Exhaustion/ Heat Cramps	No	Yes, after condition is under control.	Leave plenty of water and salt. Make sure person is comfortable. Elevate feet on rolled sleeping bag.
3	Heatstroke	No	No, unless no other way to get help.	See *Distress Signals*, p.i. Leave only after person is cooled off. Leave feet and hands in water to keep temperature down.
4	High Altitude Illness	Yes, if able to walk.	No, unless no other way to get help.	See *Distress Signals*, p.i. Set up shelter. Protect person from direct contact with ground if possible. Make sure person is comfortable. Leave fluids.

Contents

Contents